ALLERGIE

A pioneer in the field of clinical ecology
describes how environmental allergies can cause
physical illness and what can be done to identify
allergy-producing substances in our daily lives.

ALLERGIES: YOUR HIDDEN ENEMY

How the New Science of Clinical
Ecology is Unravelling the Causes of
Mental and Physical Illness

by

THERON G. RANDOLPH M.D.

and

RALPH W. MOSS Ph.D.

Foreword by Dr Richard Mackarness

THORSONS PUBLISHERS LIMITED
Wellingborough, Northamptonshire

First published in the USA by Lippincott
and Crowell, Publishers, New York

First published in the UK by Turnstone Press Limited 1981
Second Impression 1982
This edition first published 1984

British Library Cataloguing in Publication Data

Randolph, Theron G.
  Allergies: your hidden enemy
  1. Allergy
  I. Title   II. Moss, Ralph W.
  616.97   RC584

  ISBN 0-7225-0981-2

Printed and bound in Great Britain.

This book is dedicated to all patients who have ever been called neurotic, hypochondriac, hysterical, or starved for attention, while actually suffering from environmentally induced illness.

Acknowledgments

We would like to thank the following individuals for their help in the preparation of this book: Lawrence P. Ashmead, the late Ruth Hagy Brod, David and Jane Elliott, George F. Kroker, M.D., Marshall Mandell, M.D., Martha B. Moss, Janet M. (Tudy) Randolph, and John C. Wakefield, M.D. We would also like to thank the members and supporters of the Society for Clinical Ecology and the Human Ecology Action League (HEAL) for their indispensable contributions to this field.

We are also especially indebted to the directors of and contributors to the Human Ecology Research Foundations.

Contents

Foreword

On Tuesday 10 February 1981, more than two hundred doctors attended an evening meeting at the Royal College of Physicians in London, under the chairmanship of the President, Sir Douglas Black, F.R.C.P., to hear Professor M. H. Lessof from Guy's Hospital and Dr M. L. Clark from St Bartholomew's, speak on food allergies and answer the question, 'Are they fact or fantasy?' In his summary, Dr Clark said: 'There seems little doubt that food allergy exists', and both he and Professor Lessof emphasized the need for accurate diagnosis.

That such a meeting could be held at all, let alone in such a prestigious place and organized by top members of the medical establishment in Britain, is due largely to the pioneering work of one man — Dr Theron Randolph, author of this remarkable book.

For over fifty years, during the last twenty-five of which I have been privileged to know him, Ted Randolph has battled to get allergy to common foods and chemicals recognized as a major cause of human ills. He would be forgiven a smile of satisfaction had he been at that meeting at the Royal College.

This book is the first Dr Randolph has directed at the general public, after a lifetime of publishing his findings for the medical profession. Wisely, I think, he has enlisted the help of Ralph Moss, an experienced journalist, to put his ideas across in clear, non-technical language. The result is a book which must rank as a landmark in popular medical literature, coming as it does, from the man who, more than any other doctor, is turning the medical profession away from aggressive drugging, high technology and last-ditch surgery, back to whole-person medical practice.

Randolph's great contribution has been to show that what twentieth-century man has done and is doing to the environment, including food, drink and air, is responsible for at least 30 per cent of the sickness which takes people to the doctor. His treatment for food allergy is now being accepted by the medical profession and it is timely for him to explain it to the suffering public. Even more important, in the long run, is his work on the chemical hazards to health in our modern, industrialized society.

He first wrote this up for doctors in his book *Human Ecology and Susceptibility to the Chemical Environment,** which has become a classic and has been reprinted seven times. Allergy, or failure of adaptation, to the common contaminants of indoor air, including the fumes of cigarettes, gas and oil-burning appliances, has been shown by Randolph and his colleagues to be a common cause of a host of mysterious complaints for which our National Health Service provides little effective treatment: migraine, colitis, muscle and joint pains, day-long fatigue, depression, panic attacks and many other symptoms disabling urban people, symptoms for which surgical operations and more and more drugs can do little.

So ineffective has modern medical treatment become, that few people now take notice of what doctors say. Surveys on patients given drugs by their doctors have shown that as many as 50 per cent do not swallow the pills prescribed. 'Keep taking the tablets' has become a sick joke at the expense of the medical profession.

In fact, the three main forms of treatment available under the N.H.S. at vast and ever-increasing cost to the taxpayer—operations (for things like hernia and accidental injury) technology (kidney machines, cardiac pacemakers, etc.) and drugs with specific actions (antibiotics for pneumonia, analgesics and anaesthetics for pain)—cover only about 20 per cent of modern sickness.

The other 80 per cent get fobbed off with prescriptions for fairly useless drugs, the action of which the doctor does not fully understand, or, in the last report, referral to a psychiatrist, on the assumption that the symptoms complained of are all in the mind.

In its more thoughtful moments, the medical profession is aware of this alarming situation and it was admitted in a recent editorial in the *British Medical Journal* (10 November, 1979): 'In the case of much treatment with antibiotics and psychotropic drugs (drugs affecting the mind), we know virtually nothing; not the optimum dose, nor the frequency, not the duration of treatment.' Yet the annual N.H.S. drug bill is now running at £760 *million*!

Readers of this book will find an answer to this acute dilemma of the Health Service. By applying what Dr Randolph has to say, many of you will, I predict, learn how to become well and stay well with nothing more expensive than a change of diet or turning off the gas taps in your homes.

RICHARD MACKARNESS, M.B., B.S., D.P.M.
Clinical Ecology Research Unit,
Basingstoke District Hospital,
Hampshire.

office, I had to excuse myself. I walked briskly to downtown Chicago, valiantly bypassing dozens of restaurants where coffee pots steamed on their burners or shoppers lifted their cups enticingly. I needed a fix! Just when I thought I had the problem licked, I walked past a French-style cafe in the Water Tower shopping complex. The odor of fresh ground coffee wafted out at me, and it was not long before I was seated before a big, hot mug of delicious java.

Before I could finish the cup, however, a headache, like a point of pressure in either temple, had started up. In addition, my heart began to flutter like a butterfly. I was astounded, for these were my two major medical problems. Frequent headaches, especially upon arising, had been with me since—well, since I had started drinking coffee, twenty years before. The worrisome, butterfly-like palpitations had begun more recently, a few weeks earlier. I later realized that the palpitations had begun just after I had doubled my coffee intake on the quick-weight-loss diet.

I returned to the Randolphs' apartment, fighting off the surging pain in my head. I struggled through dinner, distracting the pressure with interesting conversation, and finally announced that I was going to bed. I could not sleep, however. After several more hours the headache had become so intense that I had to tie a leather belt around my temples to keep my head from flying apart, or so it felt. The Randolphs had gone to sleep, and I rambled around the apartment looking high and low for an aspirin or pain-killer.

Aspirin was what I always resorted to when I got a headache, but this time I was out of luck. The Randolphs do not own any aspirin or any other pain-killers. In fact, I could find no drugs whatsoever. A doctor without drugs seemed like a crime against nature! Never had I felt such pain as this "cold turkey" treatment for my coffee headache. I could neither lie down nor get up, stay in the darkness nor stand the light; even the tiny nightlight seered my eyeballs. I had simply never had to go the whole distance with my headache before, and I had not been aware of just how bad this problem had become. I had always been able to turn it off with those handy little white tablets.

After that experience, I stayed away from coffee for several months— more or less. On the few occasions on which I tried to drink it again, the headache and palpitations returned. After six months or so, I was able to resume drinking decaffeinated coffee, but only once every four days, according to the principles of the Rotary Diversified Diet, which will be explained later.

I do not get palpitations any more unless I drink coffee or consume other beverages, such as tea, cola, or chocolate, which contain caffeine or similar alkaloids. I rarely get headaches any more, which is remarkable, since I used to have them several times a week. They had become so common that I had grown to accept them as a permanent feature of my life and erroneously attributed them to "using my eyes too much." This was nonsense; the problem mainly was coffee.

There are those, of course, who will say that my recovery had a psychological basis and who are willing to provide free analyses of my mental state to support their argument. I do not believe this in my own case, nor do I believe it of the vast majority of the patients whom I have met, read about, and discussed. Food allergy is real. Unlike some "fashionable" ideas of psychiatry, Randolph's theories are demonstrable, provable through simple tests, and subject to the scientific benchmark of *causality*, which the dictionary defines as the principle that "nothing can exist or happen without a cause."

The concern to demonstrate cause and effect is one of the cornerstones of Randolph's thinking, and it places him in the mainstream of medical thinking of the last one hundred years. The overall course of modern medicine has been characterized by an increasing ability to demonstrate cause and effect. Until the nineteenth century, in general, physicians could only explain *what* was effective. With the development of anatomy, physiology, and related biological sciences, physicians began to explain *why*.

The discovery of the germ theory of disease by Pasteur, Koch, and others seemed to unlock the secrets of illness. Strict, uniform rules were set down for determining the exact cause of an infectious disease. Every illness from leprosy to tuberculosis, from carbuncles to dysentery, was reinterpreted in terms of its possible microbial origin. What was sometimes missing in this enthusiasm was the equally important rule played by the individual in resisting disease.

The concept of illness as an interaction between an external factor and an internal capacity for resistance did not emerge until the end of the nineteenth century and the beginning of the twentieth. The science of immunology took into account this individualized response to external factors. An equally profound advance was made by the Austrian pediatrician, Clemens von Pirquet, who coined the term "allergy" in 1906. This term was derived from two Greek words and meant "altered reactivity." An "allergy" was literally a response to a substance which affected one person but not another. It was a personal reaction to some common, nontoxic substance. Pollen, for example, caused reactions in some people, but was harmless to most. Lucretius had expressed the same idea poetically 2,000 years previously: "One man's meat is another man's poison" (Ut quod ali cibus est aliis fuat acre venenum). Von Pirquet and the other pioneers of allergy put such observations on a more scientific basis.

The field of allergy flourished, and scientists began to extend the basic concepts to various aspects of the environment, including food. (Allergy-like reactions to uncommon foods, such as cashews or shell fish, were known to the ancient Greeks.) At the turn of the century, in fact, Francis Hare, an Australian physician, wrote a massive two-volume work on *The Food Factor in Disease* (1905). In it, he detailed numerous cases in which common ailments, including apparent "mental" problems, were caused by eating common foods. In 1912, a New York pediatrician had diagnosed an allergy to eggs in a child, the first time in modern medicine that a common food had been linked specifically to allergy. In the 1920s, Albert Rowe published his first observations on how to eliminate suspected foods from the diet in order to detect allergies to them.

In 1925, however, as the field began to burgeon and become respectable, European allergists prevailed upon their American counterparts to restrict the definition of allergy to bodily mechanisms of reaction: in other words, allergy would now be explained solely in terms of immunologic theory. Allergies had previously been described rather loosely as "altered reactions occurring with time," a definition which left room for the new phenomena, such as food allergies, then first being observed. But after 1925, allergies were defined in terms of reactions between antigens and antibodies in the body, similar to the reactions which occur in some infections.

This new definition made the field of allergy admirably "scientific," in the narrow sense, since antibodies could be measured with ever-increasing precision. But with this decree, the allergists ruled out many bizarre and puzzling reactions which formerly had been a valid subject for inquiry. From this point forward, allergists were divided into two camps, the "orthodox," who accepted the antigen-antibody definition and worked within its boundaries, and the "unorthodox," who continued to investigate reactions in which such immunological reactions could not necessarily be demonstrated. One prominent scientist, Dr. Arthur F. Coca, of Cornell University, who was considered the dean of American immunologists, raised his voice to complain about the restriction of the field. Most other American allergists went along with the new definition.

The investigations of the food allergists—the "unorthodox" ones—became a kind of undercurrent within the profession, a heresy which was tolerated so long as it was kept in check. Complicated economic and political factors also came into play, which were beyond the control of any of the participants in this drama. Orthodox allergists focussed their attention on pollens, dusts, molds, and danders, which can produce dramatic and measurable reactions in sensitive individuals. But pollens and dusts are politically innocuous; one can criticize them as much as one likes, with few repercussions. Foods, however, especially the common ones, form the basis of powerful, interlocking financial interests. To name corn, wheat, milk, eggs, beet and cane sugar as the sources of illness, even in a minority of the population, will not make many friends among the commercial producers of these foods.

This was the situation in the field of allergy when Theron G. Randolph began his practice of medicine. He was graduated from the University of Michigan Medical School in 1933 and after four more years of training in internal medicine at Michigan, he studied for two years on a fellowship at Harvard

University and the Massachusetts General Hospital, in Boston, specializing in allergy and immunology. After practicing for three years in Milwaukee, Wisconsin, where he founded the Allergy Clinic in the Milwaukee Children's Hospital, he returned to Ann Arbor, Michigan, to become chief of the Allergy Clinic at the University of Michigan Medical School in July 1942. In 1944, Randolph was board-certified in internal medicine and in the following year he was subcertified in allergy. In July, 1944, he began the private practice of allergy on a fulltime basis in Chicago and became a member of the staff of Northwestern University Medical School, with admitting privileges at two of its affiliated hospitals.

The practice of medicine in the Chicago area was, and is, dominated by the faculties of its six medical schools and by the American Medical Association, whose national headquarters is in that city. The allergists of Chicago were solidly orthodox immunologists. Randolph boldly announced that he did not use the familiar skin tests favored by the orthodox, but concentrated on food ingestion tests. This created a stir among the physicians at the medical school. When Randolph made his morning rounds, for instance, some medical students asked to accompany him and hear his diagnoses and suggestions. His quiet, dignified pedagogic manner attracted inquisitive students. His rounds involved the students in a quest to discover the demonstrable cause of an illness in the patient's environment. Common foods were found to be the most frequent precipitating factors in these illnesses, Randolph taught, but their effects were masked. It was the physician's job to unmask "nature's medical coverup" and to teach patients to avoid those foods which were responsible for their symptoms. This approach was in sharp contrast to the usual medical school instruction at the time. Students began to challenge their professors with, "but Dr. Randolph says. . . ." The heresy was spreading.

By 1949, Randolph had begun to write copiously and to publish his views on food allergy in medical journals. In that year, he obtained an appointment to testify in the Food and Drug Administration's bread hearings in Washington, D.C.[1] Randolph requested that food ingredients, especially corn and cane and beet sugar, be listed on the labels of processed food products. His testimony, however, was negated by several other allergists who had been brought there for this purpose. Shortly after Randolph returned to Chicago, he was no longer allowed to mention his medical school affiliation in his articles; he was soon deprived of his position at Northwestern University Medical School and of his hospital privileges at Northwestern-affiliated hospitals. A major food manufacturer suddenly cancelled his research grant, which had previously been approved for extension.

Few colleagues supported him against this blatant expression of medical McCarthyism. One of those who did was Dr. George E. Shambaugh, Jr., a prominent ear-nose-and-throat specialist. Writing in the *Archives of Otolaryngology*, an American Medical Association publication, Shambaugh deplored the dismissal of Randolph for allegedly being "a pernicious influence on medical students" (the actual charge made against him). He then went on to praise Randolph for his "brilliant and original" contributions to ear-nose-and-throat medicine in our time.

Shambaugh compared Randolph to the great doctor Ignaz Semmelweis in the nineteenth century. "Because the ideas of Semmelweis were completely unorthodox, he found himself bitterly opposed by the conservative traditionalists, including the head of his department, and he was, literally, 'kicked off' the staff of the hospital," Shambaugh wrote. The parallel was clear.

Semmelweis had cracked under the strain of persecution and eventually went insane. Randolph weathered the storm, which included loss of a major portion of his income and private practice. He continued to treat whatever patients he could, compile records, and extend his clinical observations.

In 1951 he made what was probably his greatest discovery, and one which was to get him into even greater professional difficulties than his previous findings. After studying a number of patients, some of whom are discussed at length in this book, he came to the conclusion that man's increasing pollution of the environment with chemicals was a major source of chronic illness. By this he did not mean simply reactions to *toxic* chemicals, such as those which formed the "killer smogs" which wiped out hundreds of lives in England during the 1940s. Randolph had discovered something far more subtle, yet more profound, namely, ordinary, seemingly harmless chemicals in use in our homes, offices, and workplaces every day in "nontoxic" doses were responsible for a wide variety of mental, "emotional," and physical problems, from headache and depression to multiple muscle and joint aches and pains.

These discoveries were made ten years before Rachel Carson published *Silent Spring*, containing her forceful indictment of unrestrained use of chemical pesticides. The detailed articles which formed the basis of Randolph's book, *Human Ecology and Susceptibility to the Chemical Environment*, were published a year before Carson's popular volume; Randolph's book is, in fact, its medical counterpart.

Carson's book won her great fame and popularity; Randolph's work, on the other hand, although now in its sixth printing, is relatively unknown to the general public and to most of the medical profession.

Silent Spring, although it brought to the country's attention the dangers of the widespread use of chemical pesticides, deals only indirectly with the question of human disease. Randolph's work, on the other hand, is exclusively concerned with the effects of pollution on health. What is more, it proposed an alternative explanation and *alternative treatment* for numerous diseases, mental and physical. It thus incurred the displeasure not only of two of the most powerful industries in this country (the food and petrochemical interests) but of the medical profession as well.

It would be unreasonable to ask the medical profession to give up cherished ideas simply because a new concept is proposed. But the natural caution of a doctor, who holds lives in his hands, can easily become a blind opposition to anything new. This has been the experience of many innovators in this and previous centuries.

What is more, Randolph was proposing a simple way of diagnosing and treating a host of diseases which modern medicine is conspicuously unsuccessful in treating. In the field of problems which appear to be mental or emotional, which Randolph had first successfully treated in the late 1940s and early 1950s, the Chicago allergist offered a perfectly scientific, rational, and cogent approach—and was almost completely ignored by the psychiatric profession.

The psychiatrists remained wedded to a purely psychological approach to mental disease until about 1950. In that year, two momentous discoveries were made. On the one hand, Randolph proposed his ecologic approach to mental illness, which is described in this book. On the other hand, the first mind-altering, mood-elevating drugs which were to be used for treating psychosis were put on the market.

Randolph's methods were individualized and time-consuming for both doctor and patient. They did not rely on the sale of any drug, vitamin, or other commodity but, in fact, on the avoidance of such commodities. The pharmaceutical approach, on the other hand, was a mass-applicable program. Once a patient was told that she had a psychological problem, it was a simple matter for the physician to write a prescription and for the patient to take a tablet or be given an injection. What is more, these drugs formed the basis for a large industry, which grew from small beginnings in 1950 to a huge business. American doctors wrote 120 million tranquilizer prescriptions a year in the late 1970s, enough for 12 billion doses. Prescription tranquilizers alone earned the drug companies $650 million a year.[2]

It is hardly surprising, then, that organized medicine took the path of drugging the patient, as opposed to the more difficult but more logical path of deducing the actual environmental causes of a patient's illness and then treating the problem by eliminating these causes.

Despite opposition, Randolph managed to continue his full-time practice in allergy, run an innovative ecology unit in various hospitals, and most important, publish 350 scientific communications in this field, making contributions to the treatment and understanding of numerous diseases.

The boldness of his concepts and his obvious devotion to scientific medicine began to attract patients and other doctors who were dissatisfied with the inadequate state of assembly-line medicine. Together with a few like-minded colleagues, Randolph had struggled to little avail within the ranks of the orthodox allergy societies. Although continuing to hold membership in these societies and in the American Medical Association, Randolph and four others founded the Society for Clinical Ecology in 1965. By 1980, the society had attracted about 250 members, almost all of them medical doctors, and had begun to achieve some attention within orthodox medical circles. In both 1978 and 1979, for example, Randolph and his colleagues presented their views at the annual meetings of the American Psychiatric Association.

The Society for Clinical Ecology, representing the approach which Randolph inherited, in part developed, and greatly enriched, is a growing force within the medical field. It is appealing to doctors, for its medical theories are both logical and demonstrable—that is, they are not speculative but can be demonstrated in individually studied patients. Many of a physician's patients come with multiple symptoms, both physical and mental. Doctors are often taught in medical school that the more symptoms a patient has, the less credence should be given to any one of them, since it is assumed that many such patients are hypochondriacs and have imagined their symptoms. Randolph taught the opposite: the more symptoms a patient has, the more likely he is to be suffering from an environmentally induced disease. This new approach gave fresh hope to all people unfairly branded hypochondriacs, and to their honest physicians.

Thus, today, a growing number of doctors are being won over to the ecologic approach. Many of them either suffer from environmentally induced disease themselves or have been egged on by their patients to learn more about it. There is little doubt that as more patients learn about this scientific innovation, they will increase the demand for it from the medical system. This is bound to lead to further extensions of the concept, and of course, further struggles with orthodox rigidity. Yet it appears to be an idea whose time has come.

There is no question who the leader of this approach is. In fact, the veneration in which Randolph is held within the field of clinical ecology seems at first sight exaggerated. Practically every book and article in this new field pays tribute to his contribution. Many of the popular books written on the subject are dedicated to the Chicago physician or carry forewords and introductions by him.

Dr. Richard Mackarness, a British psychiatrist who now practices as a clinical ecologist, has called Randolph "far and away the most influential man in researching the subjects of food and chemical allergy," and dedicated his book, *Eating Dangerously*, to him "in affection and respect."

Similarly, Dr. Marshall Mandell dedicated his recent popular volume on clinical ecology "to you, Dr. Theron Randolph, for showing us the way." He added:

Through your efforts, each of us has a greater understanding of physical, mental and psychosomatic illness. Through your genius, we have all become much more effective members of the healing arts.

Doris J. Rapp, M.D., a Buffalo, New York, pediatric allergist, spoke for many of her colleagues when she wrote Randolph:

You are without a doubt the most exceptional and outstanding physician in the entire field of allergy. Your tremendous contributions as a medical scholar and teacher will live on forever. Your vision, foresight and dedication—in the face of *unjustified adversity*—is unequalled. You have always put "what's right" ahead of what's acceptable, established and politically expedient. Your total refusal to compromise with less than truth or fact is appreciated by all of us.

The reader will probably be curious to know something about Dr. Randolph as a man and a working physician. One of the things that immediately struck me—and made me suspicious—before I got to know him was precisely this reverent attitude of other doctors and patients. It seemed almost idolatrous.

After living with the Randolphs and getting to know both Ted and his wife, Tudy, I achieved a much better understanding of this attitude. One secret of his success has been to be human and democratic in his approach to patients. For instance, Randolph is always busy but never rushed and will spend hours teaching his patients about the ecologic approach to medicine. I think that being a patient in the Ecology Unit (Randolph's special treatment facility) must be a great educational experience, since the staff he has gathered around him shares the attitude of their mentor and conveys it to the patients as well.

One of the most unusual features of Randolph's work is his method of taking medical histories. A patient who has tried many doctors immediately senses that Randolph's way of taking notes is different from that of almost any doctor he is likely to have encountered. For Randolph practices medicine on the typewriter. The patient is ushered into his booklined office, and although the doctor is courteous and respectful, there is little in the way of preliminaries or bedside mannerisms. Randolph simply sits the patient down by his cluttered desk and proceeds to ask detailed, and often surprising, questions about the patient's past medical problems and current complaints.

Sometimes these questions may appear to have little relevance to the current malaise. For example, Randolph will ask a woman who is seeking treatment for depression about the onset of her arthritis twenty years before. When exactly did this joint pain begin? Can she associate it with some change in her life? Did she move into a new house at that time? What sort of heating system did the house have? Where was the garage located? and so forth. The patient is not certain about the connection between the arthritis and the depression, or between either of these and her garage, but she cooperates because the doctor seems to know so surely what he is doing.

Accompanied by the clickety-clack of his old-fashioned manual typewriter, Randolph builds up a picture of the patient's history quite unlike the summary statements found in most patients' medical records.

One could compare this intensive interrogation to the first session with a psychiatrist. But Randolph's attitude is basically the opposite of a psychiatrist's. He writes down what the patient tells him, no matter how bizarre the statement or complaint may seem. If the patient says that drinking water—all water—makes her sick, Randolph asked about the source of the water, the process of treatment employed in the patient's town, the frequency of mosquito abatement spraying in the neighborhood, as well as differences in the patient's reactions to water in other cities. A psychiatrist is more likely to inquire about the patient's associations with the word "water." Randolph's interest is in the physical environment, for it is here that he believes the cause and the solution are most likely to be found.

However, Randolph is not a stranger to evaluating the role of psychological factors in illness, having majored in psychology when a student at Hillsdale College in Michigan. Indeed, in his senior year there he was placed in charge of the psychology laboratory and received a faculty salary. As far as is known, his course was one of the first laboratory courses given for credit in this field in any educational institution. Because of his interest in abnormal psychology, he went on to medical school, but finding psychiatry a very imprecise science at that time (1929–1933), he went into internal medicine instead and, subsequently, allergy and clinical ecology.

Both the psychiatrist and the clinical ecologist believe that the ultimate cause of a patient's problem is hidden and must be unveiled through an intensive investigation. But for the psychiatrist, the interview itself is often part of the treatment. For clinical ecologists such as Randolph, the interview is only a prelude to the demonstration of cause and effect. The goal of his therapy is to make chronic symptoms disappear and then to bring them on, in an acute form, through a sudden reexposure, thus demonstrating their cause. This ability to make symptoms disappear and to summon them back at will often makes Randolph's method more convincing than psychotherapy, and leads the patient to understand and, hopefully, to control his problem.

Randolph's typewriter interviewing keeps him from developing the kind of mass-production techniques which have become so common among conventional allergists: for him, every patient is unique, as is the solution to each patient's problem. Through this approach he has gathered one of the most impressive collections of medical data in any private practice in the United States. A wall of filing cabinets holds the thousands of cases which Randolph has studied and recorded. Each is numbered and carefully indexed. In 1979, the Society for Clinical Ecology decided to computerize these records and the files of other doctors in the field, so that future generations can have ready access to this invaluable wealth of careful observation.

For the individual, suffering patient, however, Randolph's method of interviewing is the first indication that at last he has found someone who believes him and who seems to know how to go about solving a growing, desperate health problem.

A standard comment of Dr. Randolph's critics is to claim that while there is no reason to doubt his sincerity, nor the accuracy of his observations, many, if not all, of the reactions he observes can be equally well explained on the basis of suggestibility. The patient desperately wants to get better, they say, and to find an incriminating cause of his ailment. The doctor and his staff equally want the patient to get well. The suggestible patient therefore produces the very symptoms which he or she knows are expected, and this is recorded as a "reaction" to a food or chemical.

In conjunction with this argument, Randolph is sometimes castigated for not conducting "double blind" studies, in which some patients are given inert placebo substances, while others are given incriminated foods.

Some of these charges will be dealt with in the course of this book. I would like to forewarn the reader, however, by pointing out several facts in this case.

First of all, Dr. Randolph and some of his colleagues *have* carried out "blind" experiments on allergy patients, with results which confirm their less controlled observations. These tests have been published and recorded on film, and make fascinating viewing. My own conviction that food allergy was indeed real came from viewing such a film, produced by Dr. Doris Rapp of Buffalo, New York, at a 1978 meeting of the Society for Clinical Ecology. Dr. Rapp's patient was a little girl, who went into a catatonic state when she was given a test of scallops. The girl did not know when she was receiving the scallops and when she was getting some unincriminated food.[3]

Most of those who make this accusation against clinical ecology do so out of ignorance of the actual record of the new discipline in this regard.

In most cases, it is true, Randolph's treatment procedures are not conducted blindly. This is because he is a private practitioner, providing a service for his patients, and not a laboratory scientist or an investigator working in a well-financed research center. It is unreasonable to demand that clinical practitioners behave as if they were laboratory scientists. They cannot do so. To dismiss the careful and honest observations of such doctors, however, is to negate one of the most fruitful sources of scientific knowledge. Where would we be if we eliminated such observations from medicine? From Hippocrates and Galen to Lind, Semmelweis, or Jenner, it has been the case study, as much as anything else, which has goaded medicine forward.

Behind these objections to Randolph's method, however, one senses something deeper: a philosophical antagonism. What Randolph is saying, in effect, is *trust the patient*. The patient is not a liar, a braggart, or a fool. He usually is, in the doctor's words, an "experienced medical shopper" by necessity. Those who constantly harp on so-called placebo effects, on "hospitalitis," on "thick file cases" and "Baron Munchhausen complexes" betray a fundamental distrust of this medical consumer. Randolph, on the other hand, has developed a rapport with these patients, but sometimes at the expense of rapport with his colleagues.

Of course, whenever a major therapeutic discovery is made in medicine, there is a tendency to be overly enthusiastic and to try to apply the treatment to every conceivable case. The proponent is then accused of offering a "panacea"—one of the most pejorative terms in the medical lexicon. This tendency is increased tenfold when the new discovery is unfairly attacked.

The only way to know the ultimate value of clinical ecology to so-called mental, emotional, or physical ailments is to try this method. It will not cure every case of headache, depression, arthritis, or chronic fatigue. But both physicians and patients will find that a surprising number of ailments are, in fact, caused by unsuspected environmental factors, especially common foods and "safe" chemicals.

Whenever this realization becomes general knowledge, it will be Theron G. Randolph, more than any other individual, who will receive credit for this major contribution to modern medicine.

I
THE BASIC CONCEPTS

1
Hidden Addictions

This book offers a new approach to mental and physical health. It shows how our physical environment can be responsible for a wide range of ills, from fatigue to headaches, from arthritis to colitis, from hyperactivity to depression. It also shows how these environmentally related problems can be dramatically relieved in a relatively short time without the use of drugs or harmful procedures.

This new approach is based primarily on diet. But it must be emphasized from the start that the kind of dieting advocated by clinical ecologists has nothing to do with any of the standardized, mass-applicable dietary programs you may have heard about. It does not advocate the use of any particular nutrient, vitamin, or mineral in the fight against illness. Nor does it summarily ban any food.

Rather, it explains how you or your physician can detect and eliminate those commonly encountered foods and environmental chemicals which may be responsible for *your* ill health. The emphasis here is on the word *you:* this is an individualized approach. It concerns the interaction between you and your own particular environment, which is different from anyone else's. You must discover the foods and chemicals which may be making you feel sick without your being aware of their effect. You must eliminate them from your diet and environment, or learn to control their intake, in order to get well.

For many people, of course, "allergy" primarily means reactions to such inhalants as dusts, pollens, danders, and molds. Patients with these afflictions can also be helped by the methods of clinical ecology, especially when such allergies are made worse by hidden food and chemical reactions. In this book, however, reactions to common foods and chemicals shall be emphasized, and the more serious cases at that. This is because the allergic basis of such problems as hay fever is already well known, while serious reactions to foods and chemicals are still a largely unknown territory to most people.

I have practiced this approach to illness throughout my forty-five years as an allergist in the Midwest. I have treated about 20,000 people for food allergies and related problems and have dealt with virtually every kind of chronic illness on an allergic basis. About 7,000 of these patients were primarily suffering from so-called mental problems. The majority of these patients have been helped significantly, often after conventional methods of treatment had failed. Sometimes patients have come to me with a single well-defined ailment. Typically, however, patients have been polysymptomatic, that is, they have had a long history of many problems, physical and mental, which had left them in a general state of misery. The more symptoms they accumulated, the less their doctors have believed their complaints.

Usually, neither patients nor their physicians have suspected food allergy as the root of their problem. This is because most food allergy, by its very nature, is masked and hidden. It is hidden from the patient, hidden from his or her family, and hidden from the medical profession in general. It is said that often the solution to a difficult problem is right in front of your nose, but you cannot see it. In the case of food allergy, the source of the problem is literally in front of you, in the form of some commonly eaten substance which is bringing on and perpetuating chronic symptoms.

Of course, some people do know that they are allergic to certain foods, but generally these are foods that are rarely eaten. A person who is allergic to cashews, for instance, may break out in a rash on the rare occasions when he consumes these nuts. He overcomes this problem by simply avoiding cashews, and that is generally the end of the matter.

Allergies to commonly eaten foods are not so readily detected or avoided, however. Let us say, for instance, that you developed an allergy to milk early in life. At first, this may have resulted in acute reactions, such as a rash or a cough. In time, if the allergy was not recognized and controlled, the symptoms may have become more generalized and less easily detected. Since you probably went on drinking milk or eating milk products almost every day, one day's symptoms blurred into the next day's. You developed a chronic disease, such as arthritis, migraine, or depression. It never occurred to you that your daily dose of milk was the source of the problem.

In fact, you were probably "abusing" milk. You had become a milk junkie, a milk-o-holic. It is in the nature of this problem that a sudden loss of the craved substance can cause withdrawal symptoms. Since removal of milk brought on a particularly bad attack of the symptoms, you unconsciously learned to keep yourself on a maintenance dose. Milk in the morning with cereal, milk in your coffee, yogurt for lunch, a glass of milk with your dinner, and, of course, a platter of cheese tidbits before retiring.

Milk is just mentioned as an example. In fact, any food can be abused by overeating it. If a food is eaten in any form once in three days, or more frequently, it is being abused and may become a big problem for the consumer. Since it ordinarily takes between two and three days for a meal to make its way through the digestive tract, the person in question is not free of that food before another dose is added to the stomach. Intolerance to this food may sneak up on the person who eats it after months, years, or even decades of day-in and day-out ingestion.

The chief reason these reactions to commonly eaten foods are not readily recognized is that they are part of a pattern of constant reactions in which periods of heightened stimulation may give way to periods of letdown, or "withdrawal" effects. In the beginning of the problem, eating the food has a marked, immediate stimulatory effect lasting up to several hours. Simply by eating a particular food, such as coffee, wheat, or corn, as often as necessary, this "up" effect may be maintained for a relatively long period of time. It is only when such foods are not eaten regularly that a kind of "hangover," or withdrawal reaction, occurs. Some people find, for instance, that if they sleep late on Sunday morning they wake up with a headache, which usually goes away when they eat. The reason for this is a physical need for some food, such as coffee, which is normally taken early in the morning.

Since the delayed withdrawal effects can usually be controlled by eating some form of the same food, the whole cumulative process of reaction can be called a *food addiction*. A food addiction differs only in degree of severity from a drug addiction. In all other respects, the two phenomena are remarkably similar. In fact, I have arranged both food and drug addictions in an "addiction pyramid" (Fig. 1). At the peak of this addiction pyramid are heroin and other opiates and natural drugs. These are the most highly addicting substances known. Lesser degrees of addiction can develop, however, to synthetic drugs and to combinations of foods and drugs. Coffee, which is consumed in over 100 billion doses (cups) a year in the United States is a good example of such a mixture.[1] In fact, according to experts on addiction, "Any man and any mammal will develop an addiction if certain substances are introduced into the body in sufficiently large doses for a sufficient length of time."[2]

The relationship between allergy and addiction may seem a bit complicated at first. Actually, neither of these terms perfectly fits the disease state we are talking about.

Allergy, in this book, is used in its original meaning of any individualized reaction to an environmental substance occurring in time. This would include all those symptoms, such as rashes, hives, coughs, or sniffles, which are identified in the public mind with allergies.

When a person is exposed on an infrequent basis to some substance, and has an immediate reaction to that substance, then the cause and effect of the

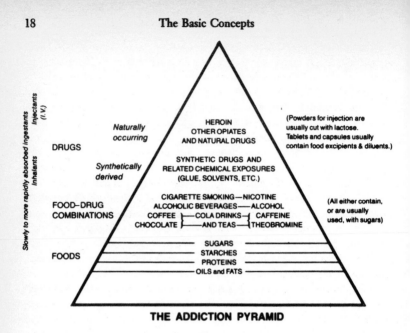

THE ADDICTION PYRAMID

allergy is apparent to all. Hay fever sufferers, for instance, have little trouble in identifying the source of their problem as pollen.

When the exposure to an allergy-causing substance is constant, however, eventually the acute symptoms will give way to either a period of no symptoms, or to chronic symptoms such as headaches, depression, or arthritis. In other words, the acute symptoms have been suppressed because of the constant nature of the exposure, and the body has reacted by attempting to adapt itself to the problem.

It is this phase which we call addiction, and this most often occurs in response to commonly eaten foods. Unlike the drug addict, however, the food addict does not usually know the object of his desire. In fact, the food addict may not consciously crave any particular food, but may simply arrange his eating schedule so that it always includes the unknown addicting substance. A milk addict, for instance, may always make himself a melted cheese sandwich before retiring, never realizing that he has a physical need for the milk product in that snack.

The food addict resembles the drug addict in one particular, however. Like the drug addict, he tends to alternate between "highs," or what we call stimulatory reactions, and "lows," which we call withdrawal reactions. Because of this alternation of "up" and "down" reactions to the addicting substance, the average person can come to understand quite well the essentially addictive nature of common food allergies.

Unfortunately, there is no single word which connotes the longing for an unknown substance, or a craving for something which is hidden not only from the world but usually from the victim himself, but the word "addiction" comes closest to that meaning.

If such food allergies are hidden, the reader may wonder how they were ever discovered. The story of their discovery by Herbert J. Rinkel, M.D., is a fascinating example of medical detective work by one of the pioneers of modern medicine.

Herb Rinkel was a technological genius, an innovator and an inventor with a passion for making cause-and-effect observations of patients and, especially, for measuring them. Under these circumstances, it is not surprising that he should come up with unusual and unique clinical observations. In my opinion, he was the outstanding clinical investigator of his day, as far as the field of allergy is concerned.[3]

Rinkel was married and had a small child when he entered Northwestern University Medical School in the 1920s. Since they had little money, he and his family subsisted mainly on eggs as their principal source of protein while he was attending medical school. His father, a Kansas farmer, sent the family a gross (144) of eggs a week. From what was later learned about food allergy, it is not surprising that under these circumstances he became highly sensitive to eggs. About this time, he developed a severe nasal allergy. Although he consulted several different physicians, the cause of his profuse rhinorrhea (running nose) was not determined, and treatment was ineffective.

Finding that the medical profession could do nothing for his nasal problem and being familiar with the early investigations of food allergy, he wondered if he might have such an allergy. However, when he tested himself with eggs by drinking down six raw eggs prepared in a blender, he failed to develop any evidence of a reaction. Several years later, however, he happened to avoid eggs along with several other foods, while testing the assumption that a combination of foods might be involved. After eliminating eggs in all forms from his diet for about five days, he ate a piece of angel food cake at a birthday party. Within a few minutes he lapsed into a state of profound physical collapse. Other physicians present were at a complete loss to explain it. Pulse, blood pressure, respiratory rate, neurological and other findings were within normal limits; unconsciousness was his only symptom. The other physicians, as well as Rinkel, after he had regained consciousness within a few minutes, were astounded by this sequence of events.

In thinking about his experience, Rinkel wondered if it might indicate something of importance about the basic nature of food allergy. Perhaps if one had been eating a given food every day, or frequently and regularly, and then omitted it for a period of several days, reexposure might induce an acute, violent type of reaction. To put this concept to the test, he began eating eggs again as formerly. He then omitted eggs again for five days, repeated the egg ingestion, and experienced another bout of unconsciousness.

Rinkel next began experimenting with several unsatisfactorily treated, chronically ill patients from the clinic where he worked. By 1936, he had confirmed and extended his observations of masked food allergy. Although these findings were reported in several local allergy journals, his major article on masked food allergy was not accepted for publication by the editor of the prestigious *Journal of Allergy*. Rinkel was very upset by this rejection and made no further attempt to publish on this subject for the following eight years. During this time he worked out the basic nature of masked and unmasked food allergy.

What foods did Rinkel and others find caused such hidden allergies? The most common culprits, quite logically, were the most commonly eaten foods. In North America at this time these include coffee, corn, wheat, milk, eggs, yeast, beef, and pork. In fact, *any* food, eaten repeatedly, could cause allergic reactions. If a person did not eat one of these foods, the chances are he would not become allergic to it. On the other hand, if a food were taken more than once every three or four days (and most of those on the above list are), then they may possibly cause trouble.

Americans have become largely unaware of what goes into their stomachs. The increased consumption of prepared food, including restaurant food, often leads us to eat blindly. Many people still do not read labels, and labels are often incomplete or inaccurate. Some labels, for example, list "sugar" as an ingredient, but rarely say whether this means cane, beet, or corn sugar.

The result of this situation is that many people think they are not consuming a particular food, when they are in fact having it every day. A good example is corn: you may not eat corn as a vegetable very often, yet eat it at practically every meal in the form of corn sugar (dextrose or glucose), corn syrup, cornstarch, corn oil, or as a hidden ingredient in other foods, such as beer or whisky. Both Rinkel and I showed that allergy to corn was, in fact, a dominant form of food allergy in North America.

In this book, therefore, when I speak of "eating" a food, I am referring to consumption of that food in any form in which it enters the body, not just in its most obvious shape. Part of the difficulty in unmasking food allergy stems from the hidden way in which various foods enter the diet.

As I have indicated, the continuous intake of such a food may eventually result in a response which resembles addiction: one has an unconscious need to consume a particular substance in order to feel relatively well. Being deprived of that substance brings on a feeling of illness, whose nature depends on the individual in question. The American humorist Don Marquis once said that "ours is a world where people don't know what they want and are willing to go through hell to get it." This is a good description of the food addict, who doesn't know the exact nature of the food he craves, but is willing to eat compulsively, to the point of addiction, in order to get it.

The addictive response is broadly composed of two phases: 1) an immediate improvement of chronic symptoms of illness, such as tiredness, headache, fatigue, or aches and pains, when the food is eaten and then 2) a delayed hangover unless the addicting food or drink is taken on schedule. Each individual establishes his own addiction routine, his own pattern of ever-decreasing periods between food "fixes." By taking his addicting food, the addict keeps himself in a relatively "high" state and postpones feelings of letdown, hangover, or pain which follow withdrawal of the addicting food.

Since the craved food results in pleasure or at least the absence of pain when it is eaten, the confirmed "food-a-holic" may indignantly reject the suggestion that his "favorite" food or drink is bad for him. Why, that's the very food that makes him feel good! This is part of the paradoxical nature of food allergy—that one's best friend, foodwise, often turns out to be one's worst enemy.

CASE STUDY: MENTAL EXHAUSTION WITH PHYSICAL FATIGUE

Charles Henderson,[4] a prominent businessman, came to see me because he was troubled by mental exhaustion, mental confusion, and fatigue. He was a top executive of a large company who dictated to a battery of secretaries from morning to night. One of his secretaries pointed out to him that he did not give understandable dictation during the late afternoon. This was hard for her, for Henderson usually scolded her the next day for not accurately reproducing his previous day's dictation.

In desperation, the secretary suggested that Henderson relax with the office staff in the afternoon and have a snack. Once he did so she was able to comprehend his words and directions somewhat better. For this man, a snack meant only one thing: eggs. In fact, he had eggs for breakfast, egg salad for lunch, and some dessert containing eggs at dinner almost every day. His secretary literally "egged him on" to have eggs at break time, as well.

When I finished taking this man's history I told him, "Mr. Henderson, I think you are allergic to eggs."

He jumped from his chair and said, "Doctor, you obviously didn't understand what I just told you! Let me repeat it: eggs are the one food I *know* agrees with me. Now you tell me I may be allergic to them. That doesn't make any sense to me at all." He was clearly on the point of walking out of the office. He knew what he was allergic to and what he wasn't.

This episode took place in the late 1940s. I had just finished a rather intensive study of drug addiction and had privately reached the conclusion that food allergy and drug addiction were aspects of the same problem. I decided to explain the problem to Henderson in terms of addiction. I explained that he seemed to have a three-hour "high" from eggs, after which he started to come down, with attendant symptoms of confusion and fatigue. He had to eat eggs every three hours or so in order to remain "high."

This made some sense to him, and he agreed to take a test to prove its validity. Since it takes between two and three days to clear any particular meal from the intestines, Henderson ate no eggs, or product containing eggs, during the next few days. He suffered from withdrawal symptoms, and was so weak that he could not get out of bed to go to work.

He began to feel better after the eggs were entirely out of his system. Then he came back to my office, where he was fed eggs in a testing room. Within less than an hour, he had returned these eggs, through violent projectile vomiting, halfway across the room. He was terribly embarrassed, but amazed to see that his "favorite" food really did not agree with him at all.

By staying off eggs for six months or so he was able to break his addiction to them. After that, he was able to reintroduce eggs into his diet, but only once every four days, in order to prevent the addiction from reforming. By controlling this and other food allergies, he was able to restore his ability to think and dictate clearly.

Henderson's case is fairly typical of food allergies in general. The man had multiple symptoms, including some which are vaguely called "mental" problems. Yet they were not "mental," in the usual sense of that term: they stemmed from actual, physical exposures, and not from psychological conflicts.

The basis of the problem lay hidden from sight and could not be readily deduced by the patient himself. In fact, common sense had led him to believe that eggs relieved his symptoms, when, in fact, they caused them.

The relationship between eggs and Henderson's fatigue was suspected on the basis of his history, but it was demonstrated by an actual feeding test, a procedure which will be described more fully later.

One should not conclude from this story that eggs, in and of themselves, are somehow particularly addicting and dangerous. One could substitute any commonly eaten food, or combination of foods, in this story, and it would still be realistic.

Food allergy is the result of an interaction between an individual and his own particular environment. Whether or not a person actually develops a food allergy depends, first of all, on his *ability to react*. Anyone can develop such an ability, but people with a family history of allergy have a greater chance of becoming sick in this way. If a patient tells me that he suffers from hay fever, for example, or that one or both of his parents does, I am more likely to suspect the existence of food allergies in his case. But a lack of overt allergies is no guarantee that the person cannot develop hidden food allergies.

Second, the development of such allergies depends on exposure. The more frequently a person is exposed to a food, the greater is his tendency to become addicted. An unusual, massive exposure can also trigger a susceptibility problem. Some patients, for example, appear able to tolerate wheat in moderate doses. But a big spaghetti dinner might bring on obvious symptoms. As can be seen from the addiction pyramid (page 18), the most rapidly absorbed portions of food, such as sugars and alcohols, are more readily addicting than more slowly absorbed foods.

Even more addicting than foods per se are food-drug combinations. These include alcoholic beverages, which are mixtures of ethyl alcohol and various food fractions. Alcoholism is, in a sense, the acme of the food-addiction problem (see Chap. 10). Coffee is a natural combination of a food (the coffee bean) and a drug—caffeine. Some kinds of coffee contain 2.5 percent caffeine. Chocolate, cola drinks, and tea are similar food-drug mixtures.

Despite the fact that our culture treats these beverages as harmless foods, many researchers now consider them to be potentially harmful mixtures of food and drugs. Caffeine, even in modest amounts (a few cupfuls of tea or coffee), can affect the heart rate, heart rhythm, blood-vessel diameter, coronary circulation, blood pressure, urination, and other bodily functions.[5] Knowing the billions of doses in which these substances are taken and the often compulsive way in which people crave their favorite beverage, one begins to suspect the existence of a widescale food-addiction problem in the United States.

Other environmental factors which may cause addictions include tobacco, drugs, and environmental chemicals. All of these may have a cumulative effect. Pollens, dusts, molds, danders, and other inhaled substances are less apt to be associated with addictive responses because exposure to them is seasonal or intermittent.

It is natural to want to know how common these food allergies or addictions are. In my experience, food allergy is one of the greatest health problems in our country. Combined with the chemical-susceptibility problem, which is discussed later, it is a growing source of ill health and particularly of those chronic, vaguely defined problems which almost never respond to conventional medical treatment.

Marshall Mandell, M.D., author of a recent book on allergies, has estimated that "50 to 80 percent of the daily medical practice of many doctors" is the result of allergy and chemical susceptibility.[6] The late Dr. Arthur Coca believed that as many as 90 percent of all Americans had one or more food allergies.[7]

Many of the people reading this book are probably suffering from some form of these problems; and the majority of their chronic illnesses which do not respond well to conventional therapy are probably caused by some undiagnosed allergy or susceptibility.

Allergies and "Mental" Problems

Allergies can not only cause familiar physical symptoms but can also be responsible for a host of so-called mental problems, including some cases of what looks like outright psychoses. Remarkably, the complete avoidance of a particular food or foods sometimes brings relief of such symptoms, while the reintroduction of the incriminating food can bring back the "mental" problem.

I first observed a possible link between food allergy and mental-behavioral problems in the late 1940s. As previously mentioned, I started performing food ingestion tests in my office upon beginning my practice in Chicago in mid-1944. A commonly eaten food to be tested would be avoided completely between four and six days before such an ingestion test. Although minor abnormalities of mood and behavior had been observed earlier in patients undergoing these tests, the following cases confirmed the credibility of the relationship between given foods and mental reactions.

CASE STUDY: HEADACHE WITH FATIGUE

Janet Cott, a young woman, complained of headache, fatigue, depression, and intermittent lapses of memory. She had been in the habit of eating eggs for breakfast for many years. After avoiding eggs for a week, she came to my office for an egg ingestion test. Five minutes after eating two eggs, she reported the onset of dizziness, heavyheadedness, and nasal stuffiness. At 10 minutes she started pacing in the food test room. At 15 minutes she began to cry in front of the other patients.

I urged her to come to another room. She either failed to understand or could not make a decision; she remained semiconscious for the following half-hour and cried intermittently for two hours. Upon recovering, she could not recall the events which had happened since the onset of the acute phase of her reaction. Her pulse rate, which had been 70 before this ingestion test, reached 104 at 30 minutes, and 110 at 60 minutes after the first feeding.

CASE STUDY: FATIGUE WITH COUGHING

A nurse, Edith Demarest, age 40, with a history of running nose, coughing, wheezing, and dizziness, later developed extreme fatigue and occasional headaches, as well as bouts of muscle-aching and depression. All symptoms were accentuated on arising in the morning but improved after drinking milk for breakfast. She also drank milk with each subsequent meal and at bedtime, never suspecting it. She improved while avoiding milk prior to a milk ingestion test. After drinking milk for the test, she developed, at 10 minutes, waves of yawning and sleepiness and then severe episodes of coughing and wheezing. A headache developed at 45 minutes and persisted for 15. At 60 minutes there was increased puffiness of her hands and eyes. The pulse rate of 68 at the start changed to 69, 72, and 76, at 20, 40, and 60 minutes. The white blood-cell count of 7,300 at the start decreased to 3,500, 2,400, and 2,200 cells at 20, 40, and 60 minutes.

Whereas this patient, a recent arrival in Chicago, had usually been timid when driving in traffic, she later admitted that she felt punch-drunk and very happy upon leaving the office two hours after drinking milk. She drove to her home with self-confidence and utter abandon, relatively oblivious to traffic hazards. An hour after arriving home, she felt increasingly hazy and less happy. After taking a short nap, she awakened crying and complained of intense headache, associated with pains across her shoulders, and continued depression. Residual effects persisted for two days. It is interesting that coughing and wheezing were absent during the time she had more cerebral symptoms, such as headache and depression.

Two weeks later, an ingestion test with milk was performed, all milk products having been avoided in the meantime. An increased sense of lightheadedness occurred at 3 minutes. This was followed by extreme sleepiness and grogginess at 5 minutes, which was associated with an inability to read comprehendingly. The patient then developed spasms of severe coughing after 8 minutes, and again at 40 minutes. Some crying occurred 5 minutes later, and sleepiness, grogginess, and persistent headache continued.

Although Mrs. Demarest reported feeling fine at the end of two hours, she again became pale, dopey, and sleepy upon reaching home three hours after the start of the test. The next morning she still had a slight residual headache.

CASE STUDY: HEADACHE WITH FATIGUE AND DEPRESSION

Another woman patient, Ida Koller, age 24, had complained of headaches associated with fatigue and intermittent periods of depression. I noticed that she was slightly dizzy and more talkative than formerly following a milk test in the office, but she assured me that she felt fine and was able to drive home.

Approximately one hour later, I received a telephone call from a suburban police department that Miss Koller had been arrested for "drunken driving."

She gave the unlikely story that all she had had to drink was a glass of milk in her doctor's office. Since she did not have any odor of alcohol on her breath, the police were puzzled and called me; I confirmed her story. When asked to state this in writing, I complied, and explained how acute allergic reactions to foods may simulate alcoholic inebriation.

Clinical observations of this type which I made in the late 1940s opened several promising avenues for medical investigation, with the following tentative deductions:

1. Chronic reactions to the cumulative intake of given foods (best referred to as food addictions) occur initially as stimulatory levels of reaction, but later show up as progressive withdrawal responses (see Chap. 2).
2. Acute reactions to a food (in a food ingestion test) compress the stimulatory-withdrawal sequence into a time frame of minutes or hours in a manner which can be compared to time-lapse photography; this exaggerates the severity of both phases.
3. Alcoholic beverages and sugars prepared from given foods, because of their greatly increased rate of absorption, induce both chronic and acute reactions more readily than do more slowly absorbed forms of the same food.

These tentative deductions were confirmed and extended by additional clinical observations. My cumulative clinical experience led to the correct interpretation of events in the most advanced case of allergy with "mental" symptoms which I had seen up to that time, the case of Mary Hollister.

CASE STUDY: PSYCHOSIS AND WANDERING MANIA

In 1949, Mary Hollister, age 30, was referred to me from an adjacent state with the complaint of incapacitatingly severe headaches. In some of the more serious episodes of her illness, she drifted into periods of extreme hyperactivity which resembled the effects of alcoholism, even though she had not drunk any alcoholic beverage. These episodes were followed by severe depression. Upon recovering from these acute bouts, Mrs. Hollister had no memory of the events which had transpired during them.

When first seen in my office, Mrs. Hollister was too confused to provide an adequate history. Thinking that she was too ill to be handled on an outpatient basis, I decided to have her hospitalized and placed on an elimination diet which avoided several major foods. When visited in the hospital later the same day, she was drinking coffee, which was not on her diet. With the complete avoidance of coffee and other prohibited foods, she became increasingly reclusive and depressed for the next two days.

Following this withdrawal, Mrs. Hollister improved progressively and was soon leading a normal, socially well-adjusted life, going about the floor campaigning for her favorite political candidate. Able to receive a detailed history for the first time, I learned that she had been drinking approximately 40 cups of coffee daily, each cup containing two teaspoonfuls of beet sugar. The diet upon which she improved contained only cane sugar. By pure chance, it had also eliminated four other foods which were later to be incriminated as the sources of food allergies.

When I saw her during the evening meal of her sixth hospital day, I noticed that she was eating beets as a vegetable. Upon leaving the hospital, I went to a far suburb of Chicago to lecture. I had only been there for a few minutes when I received an urgent phone call from the hospital. Mary Hollister was psychotic, racing for the exits, screaming, kicking, yelling, and trying by every means to get out of the place. She was even leaning out of the eighth floor window, her nurse told me, desperately seeking to get more air and apparently unaware of the danger of falling out.

I prescribed the injection of a sedative and left instructions that if this were ineffective they were to apply physical restraints. Mrs. Hollister was sleeping when I checked with the hospital later. But when I visited her the next morning, she failed to recognize me, to remember my name, or to recall other events of the past thirteen years. As her hyperactivity gradually decreased, she became progressively depressed. Although it was possible to remove the restraints after 36 hours, she remained apathetic, extremely depressed, disoriented, and amnesic for the following 24 hours. Then suddenly, and with little advance warning, she became correctly oriented as to time, place, and person.

Seeking a possible explanation for this strange episode, I recalled that she had eaten beets in the evening meal two hours before the onset of this attack. I now suspected that beets, which she had formerly eaten—frequently in the form of beet sugar—and was then eating for the first time in six days—may have induced the reaction, although no one at the time had ever described psychosis resulting from food intake.

After this acute reaction had subsided, I obtained permission to insert a tube through her nose into her stomach for the purpose of feeding her without her knowing what food she was being given. We waited expectantly for a reaction after infusing milk, but nothing happened. However, after another "blind" infusion of beets and beet juice the next day, an identical acute reaction was induced and photographed. Again she was, to all appearances, psychotic. Yet this was the result of nothing more complicated than a test reexposure to a common food which she had previously eaten on a day-in and day-out basis. As far as can be determined from having shown a film of this incident at medical meetings in many countries, this is the first recorded instance of an advanced psychotic episode resulting from a test feeding of an allergenic food.

It should be pointed out that this case and the more briefly described instances leading up to it were extreme examples gleaned from a large clinical experience. These extreme cases stimulated interest in studying the possible role of food allergy-addiction in mental and behavioral disturbances, including less severe cases.

Mary Hollister's case is considered by many to be a landmark in the understanding of this form of psychosis and of "mental" problems in general. There are, of course, many *theories* of mental illness. Usually, however, these theories cannot be proved or disproved, and a true cause of the illness cannot be demonstrated with any degree of scientific accuracy. Mary Hollister's illness could be relieved or induced simply by manipulating her intake of particular foods—in her case, beets or beet sugar (although a few less important foods were also incriminated).

The cause of her problem remained hidden from her and her previous physicians because of the masked nature of allergies to common foods. Her constant, almost hourly, consumption of beet sugar kept her in a state of relatively normal behavior, but like any "junkie" she was always in danger of failing to get her "fix" or of getting an overdose of her addicting substance.

Mary Hollister's case raised for the first time the possibility that other forms of so-called mental problems, including the various neuroses usually handled by psychotherapy, could also have an allergic basis. In pursuing this idea over the past thirty years, I have found that food allergies and chemical susceptibility do indeed cause a wide range of "mental" and behavioral problems. In fact, in this period I have seen many problems normally treated by psychiatry successfully diagnosed and treated through the methods of clinical ecology.

These "mental" and physical problems, I discovered, do not occur at random in the life of an individual, but are part of an overall continuum of symptoms in which a patient progresses from various levels of stimulation to corresponding levels of withdrawal in a predictable way, as will be described in the following chapters.

2
The Ups and Downs of Addicted Life

The addict is basically unstable, in that he tends to require an ever-increasing dose of his addicting substance in order to keep well. By keeping "well" is meant the maintenance of immediate stimulatory effects ("highs") and avoidance of delayed withdrawal effects ("hangovers," or "lows"). This is true of the drug addict, food addict, or alcohol addict. The main difference between these types of addictions is that the drug addict usually knows the identity of his addicting substance, whereas the food addict is ordinarily hooked on one or more unrecognized foods. The drink addict, or alcoholic, is usually hooked not on alcohol per se but on one or more foods from which alcoholic beverages are derived. More will be said about addiction to these food-drug combinations later.

An addiction response is quite properly referred to as a "trip." Such a journey, consisting of many ups and downs, may stretch over many years. At first, the "highs" of addiction may be pleasant and rewarding. But as the "trip" continues, such "highs" tend to become less desirable, though still far preferable to the more disastrous "lows." The addict's prospects are bleak, whether he is hooked on foods, drink, or drugs. Generally speaking, he tends to climb to a certain stimulatory level before falling into a pit. The pit consists of increasingly common and prolonged withdrawals which can no longer be avoided or postponed by recourse to the formerly effective substances. Allergies of all sorts, including fatigue, aches and pains, and depression come to dominate the addict's life. When he is no longer able to cope with these withdrawals as he formerly could, he finally seeks medical care.

Table 1 presents the various levels of addiction and the manner in which they affect the addict's physical and mental state. It can be seen from this chart that many of the most common chronic illnesses can actually be way

Table 1. The Ups and Downs of Addiction

Directions: Start at zero (0). Read up for predominantly Stimulatory Levels; read down for predominantly Withdrawal Levels.

Maladapted Cerebral and Behavioral Responses	**+ + + +** MANIC, WITH OR WITHOUT CONVULSIONS	Distraught, excited, agitated, enraged, and panicky. Circuitous or one-track thoughts, muscle-twitching and jerking of extremities, convulsive seizures, and altered consciousness may develop.
	+ + + HYPOMANIC, TOXIC, ANXIOUS, AND EGOCENTRIC	Aggressive, loquacious, clumsy (ataxic), anxious, fearful, and apprehensive; alternating chills and flushing, ravenous hunger, excessive thirst. Giggling or pathological laughter may occur.
Adapted Responses	**+ +** HYPERACTIVE, IRRITABLE, HUNGRY, AND THIRSTY	Tense, jittery, "hopped-up," talkative, argumentative, sensitive, overly responsive, self-centered, hungry, and thirsty; flushing, sweating, and chilling may occur, as well as insomnia, alcoholism, and obesity.
	+ STIMULATED BUT RELATIVELY SYMPTOM-FREE	Active, alert, lively, responsive, and enthusiastic, with unimpaired ambition, energy, initiative, and wit. Considerate of the views and actions of others. This usually comes to be regarded as "normal" behavior.
	0 BEHAVIOR ON AN EVEN KEEL, AS IN HOMEOSTASIS	Calm, balanced, level-headed reactions. Children expect this from their parents and teachers. Parents expect this from their children. We all expect this from our associates.
Maladapted Localized Responses	**−** LOCALIZED ALLERGIC MANIFESTATIONS	Running or stuffy nose, clearing throat, coughing, wheezing. Asthma, itching (eczema and hives), gas, diarrhea, constipation (colitis), urgency and frequency of urination, and various eye and ear syndromes.
Maladapted Systemic Responses	**− −** SYSTEMIC ALLERGIC MANIFESTATIONS	Tired, dopey, somnolent, mildly depressed, edematous with painful syndromes (headache, neckache, backache, neuralgia, myalgia, myositis, arthralgia, arthritis, arteritis, chest pain), and cardiovascular effects.*
Maladapted Advanced Stimulatory Responses	**− − −** BRAIN-FAG, MILD DEPRESSION, AND DISTURBED THINKING	Confused, indecisive, moody, sad, sullen, withdrawn, or apathetic. Emotional instability and impaired attention, concentration, comprehension, and thought processes (aphasia, mental lapse, and blackouts).
	− − − − SEVERE DEPRESSION, WITH OR WITHOUT ALTERED CONSCIOUSNESS	Unresponsive, lethargic, stuporous, disoriented, melancholic, incontinent, regressive thinking, paranoid orientation, delusions, hallucinations, sometimes amnesia and coma.

* Cardiovascular manifestations, including rapid or irregular pulse, hypertension, phlebitis, anemia, and bleeding and bruising tendencies, may occur at any level.

stations of the addiction trip. These include some problems usually dismissed as "psychosomatic" by physicians and psychotherapists.

STIMULATORY REACTIONS

At birth, a person usually starts out at the zero level, which we call "behavior on an even keel." Generally speaking, he is at peace with himself. He is placid, not subject to violent squalls of mood or emotion. This is the kind of "normal" behavior which children usually expect from their parents and teachers. Parents expect it from their children. We all expect it from our co-workers, business associates, and friends. Yet how rarely we get it!

If such a placid person begins to develop an allergic type of addiction to a food or other substance, he usually enters first the plus-one (+) phase. This stage can be highly deceptive. Except for a trained observer, it is difficult for the person himself or those close to him to distinguish behavior at this stage from normal activity.

The person at the plus-one stage is active, alert, lively, responsive, and enthusiastic. He has ambition, energy, initiative, and wit. He is considerate of the views and desires of others. In time, his more or less placid personality (zero stage) is forgotten, and everyone assumes that his plus-one personality is the "real" one. It is not. Although it appears socially harmless and even desirable, this constantly stimulated stage represents a response to an addiction to an unknown substance, in its earliest form.

Medical care by a clinical ecologist at this stage could detect the source of the mildly stimulated reaction. But such a person almost never comes to a doctor. Why should he? He feels well, gets along well with those around him, and is probably quite successful at school or work. Sometimes, perhaps, his high energy level may get on the nerves of his acquaintances, but no one suspects that this is the sign of a developing disease process.

Such a person is riding the crest of mildly stimulated reactions to foods, drinks, drugs, or chemicals. His response to life situations is sustained, as are normal responses, but they are exaggerated. A salesperson, for instance, in this early plus-one phase, may hang up an enviable record, because he is active, energetic, vigorous, and even slightly aggressive. He would be amazed or incredulous if anyone suggested that he were beginning to get sick. He likes himself this way and so does his employer, for he can be highly productive; in the short run, he may be more productive than the truly normal person. His friends generally enjoy his company and enthusiasm.

It bears repeating, however, that such a person may have already developed the first stage of a potentially dangerous allergy, an addiction to some common part of the environment, such as an ever-present cup of coffee, soft drink, a cigarette, a meal which always must contain certain foods, or even the fumes and odors of traffic or of a particular place, such as an automobile showroom or garage.

If the plus-one individual maintains his addictive responses to such substances or if he adds new addictions to existing ones, he is not likely to stay at the mildly stimulated level. In time, he will probably "graduate" to a higher level of addiction, plus-two $(++)$.

At plus-two, the addictive patterns begin to be a problem for the individual and those around him. Of course, months and years may elapse between the onset of the plus-one and plus-two stages, but eventually the supersalesman may become a super problem for those around him. A person at the plus-two phase may be tense, jittery, "hopped-up," talkative, argumentative, sensitive, overly responsive, self-centered, and constantly hungry and thirsty. He may have sudden fits of flushing, sweating, and chilling.

At the plus-two level, three big health problems appear. The first of these is hyperactivity, occurring mostly in children. I first reported hyperactivity in children on the basis of food allergy in 1947 and hyperactivity from food additives and contaminants and other environmental chemicals in 1962. Dr. Benjamin Feingold and others have pointed to the role of artificial colorings and flavorings in producing hyperactivity. But this is only a small part of the picture. Children can develop addictive-allergic responses to virtually any part of their environment, including—but not limited to—artificial food additives. The seriousness of this problem is underlined by the fact that one-tenth to one-fifth of grade school children are said to be hyperactive to some degree[1] (see Chap. 9).

A second major health problem engendered at this stage is obesity. The hyperactive adult or child craves food and drink. He particularly craves those dishes or snacks which contain his addictant(s), and often calls this his "favorite food." Such an individual often needs a "fix" in order to get to sleep at night: he is an inveterate midnight refrigerator raider. He may wake up in the middle of the night and help himself to more food. Invariably, he keeps the refrigerator well stocked with his addicting items. Sometimes family members will joke that he seems to be addicted to sweets, cheese, steak, or whatever is his favorite treat. If only they knew how right they are!

Finally, plus-two is the phase at which alcoholism develops. This is because the victim craves food and drink in general, because his way of life often brings him into contact with alcohol, but especially because alcoholism is itself frequently a heightened form of food allergy. It is, in fact, the acme of food addiction, and the alcoholic in his maladapted behavior is usually reacting to the foods from which his beverage is manufactured rather than to the druglike effects of the alcohol itself. This point is amplified and explained in Chapter 10.

Our once happy and successful plus-one salesman is now less than enviable. Because of compulsive eating, he probably is somewhat paunchy, if not actually fat. He very likely drinks too much, trying to maintain the high spirits of his former plus-one personality. At home he is probably overactive, with the "restless legs" syndrome. He quarrels with his wife and children, cannot get comfortable, and has become a general nuisance to those around him. He may complain at times that he is "crawling out of his skin," but cannot explain where he wants to go or what he wants to do.

He has probably burned himself out professionally, by antagonizing his customers with a too effusive sales routine, and alienated his fellow workers and employer with his counterproductive competitiveness and aggressiveness. His once desirable enthusiasm has been carried so far that it can now be seen for what it really is—a pathological condition—and his previous success has turned into failure.

This is as "high" as most such individuals ever go. But if the plus-two individual continues to mount the stimulatory ladder, he will reach the plus-three phase (+++). At this phase he may sometimes appear to be drunk without ever having taken a drop. He is loud, talkative, clumsy, and overbearing. He may be anxious, and afraid of real or imagined dangers, or racked by alternating chills and flushing, ravenous hunger, and excessive thirst. At times, his symptoms may include giggling or pathological laughter. People think that he is quite strange and tend to stay away from him. Such individuals generally have lost all pretensions to normal behavior, and are also so self-centered that they tend to be indifferent to the aims, thoughts, and feelings of others.

Some of these people, however, can keep up a pretense of normality in certain situations. They may, at first sight, appear to be highly dynamic, charged-up leaders, who know without hesitation the way forward in any situation. They make disastrous leaders, however, for they substitute egomania and unfounded enthusiasm for sound judgment. If one becomes involved with such a person, one gradually realizes that something is basically wrong. The hopped-up person is making all the decisions, and most of them are disastrous. At this point, one is lucky if he can cut his losses and get out of the relationship without a major argument.

Finally, the plus-three individual may progress to the plus-four phase (++++). By now he is obviously a sick person; in fact, this phase is identical in appearance to the manic phase of manic-depressive disease. By this point, the increasing degree of overstimulation caused by an advanced addiction has resulted in an extreme lack of physical and mental control. The plus-four person is quite simply out of his mind, a classic case of psychosis. He flails his limbs, has convulsions, and shows other forms of extreme, irrational behavior. His thought processes are equally bizarre; he is obsessed by strange, irrational ideas, quite inappropriate to his actual situation. (Mary Hollister, in her reaction to beets, often acted like a typical plus-four patient.)

It is relatively rare, however, for an allergy patient to go higher than the plus-two phase. The addicting substance usually loses its "kick" before this, and the victim has increasingly frequent "hangovers."

Sometimes, however, the stimulated person identifies the source of his addiction and is able to resort to it in just the right dose, frequently enough, to postpone his downward slide. A person may discover, for instance, that he must have a cup of coffee every morning in order to perform his job. He may then discover that he needs another cup at noon to prevent a let-down feeling. He may then go on increasing his well-timed doses to keep himself in a state of relative "health" for the duration of the day. Eventually, such a precarious system breaks down, and the person is faced with the negative side of the addiction picture, usually after some personal health disaster has occurred.

Withdrawal Reactions

The stimulatory (plus) levels can all be considered, in a sense, adaptive responses by the body to some environmental substance(s). When the body can no longer adapt, it enters the various stages of maladaptation (see Chap. 11). These are the withdrawal reactions, also called hangovers or letdowns. Most people never identify their stimulatory (plus) reactions as symptoms until the bigger picture is pointed out to them. The negative reactions are clearly problems, however, and doctors' waiting rooms are filled with the victims of such reactions.

Minus-one reactions are those symptoms, mainly physical, which are *commonly* called allergic reactions. They include running nose, coughing, wheezing, asthma, itching, hives, eczema, excessive gas, diarrhea, constipation, colitis, and other localized physical problems.

Because such reactions are ordinarily considered as allergic in origin and handled by conventional allergists, I have given little detailed attention to them in this book. It can be assumed, however, that they are often caused by allergies to foods and common chemicals.

Minus-one reactions (−) such as these may disappear, only to be replaced by even more troublesome minus-two (−−) reactions. Minus-two reactions are "systemic" allergic symptoms, affecting not just one but many parts of the body. A person in this stage of allergy is typically tired, dopey, sleepy, or mildly depressed. He is frequently plagued by *painful* syndromes, such as headache, neckache, backache, neuralgia, myalgia, and arthralgia. This is the phase in which chest pains and cardiovascular effects are noticed. Cardiovascular ·mptoms can include rapid or irregular pulse or heartbeat, hypertension, phlebitis, anemia, or tendencies toward bleeding and bruising.

Typically these symptoms do not occur alone. That is, by the time a patient has fallen to the minus-two level, he often has many of these problems. Doctors like to deal with anatomically distinct problems: "Where does it hurt?" is a typical opening question. Few doctors like to hear, "It hurts all over," or some such reply. In fact, as we have mentioned, many doctors are told in medical school to discount the statements of patients with many complaints. For this reason, patients in the minus-two and minus-three categories are often told, condescendingly, that their problems are "all in their head," or psychosomatic. This may be due to the unfamiliarity of orthodox physicians with the findings of clinical ecology. In actuality, such multiple symptoms are often the end result of a long process of developing allergy. The individual nature of the patient's problem can usually be demonstrated through the methods of clinical ecology.

Minus-two (−−) is the stage at which we find such common problems as physical fatigue and headache (Chap. 12) and muscle and joint aches and pains, including arthritis (Chap. 13). Fatigue, when related to food allergy, tends to be worse in the morning, because this is when the patient has been without his addictant for several hours. He needs, and craves, his fix. Fatigue on an allergic basis is usually quite different from physical fatigue resulting from exertion, which is relieved by rest and sleep. Allergic fatigue is seemingly without cause, and is not ordinarily relieved by prolonged periods of rest; it is basically quite unpleasant.

Minus-three (−−−) is the stage I call "brain-fag." The term "brain-fag" is found in Webster's dictionary as a synonym for mental exhaustion. It was suggested to me by a patient who suffered from this problem, and I have used it ever since. "Brain-fag" is more than just exhaustion. In this stage, thinking is confused, and people become indecisive, moody, sad, sullen, withdrawn, or apathetic. There is frequently much emotional instability and impaired attention. The "brain-fagged" patient cannot concentrate properly, and his comprehension and thought processes are impaired. This includes aphasia (the inability to speak, or to find words for things), mental lapses, and blackouts. A fuller discussion of "brain-fag," with case histories, is given in Chapter 14.

As with the minus-two reactions, "brain-fag" is characteristically polysymptomatic. The patient has many symptoms and often has periods of physical illness (minus-one or -two) interspersed with his generalized mental exhaustion (minus-three).

Severe depression, or minus-four (−−−−), can be called the end of the line of this entire problem. This depression can be preceded by a superstimulated (plus-four) phase, as in manic-depressive disease, or by less severe withdrawal symptoms (minus-three).

While depression does occur in the young, it is most commonly found in the middle-aged or elderly, who have had a lifetime to develop to this stage. Such depression is often believed to be the result of unhappy events in the life of the patient, such as bereavement, retirement, or changes of locale. While such life events may contribute to the problem, usually mild depression and "brain-fag" precede them, and provide the underlying mechanism for the development of a crisis. Most often, in my experience, depression is caused by lifelong addictions to common foods, drinks, and environmental chemicals.

The severely depressed person may be unresponsive, lethargic, disoriented, and melancholic. While he may remain rational for long periods of time, he may eventually lapse into paranoid thinking, delusions, hallucinations, and sometimes even amnesia and coma.

The Ups and Downs of the Addiction Trip

These, then, are the basic way stations of the addiction trip. As indicated, however, there is nothing static about any of these stages; the patient moves from one to another and from stimulatory to withdrawal phases, as his problem develops. The ultimate trip, in this regard, is the progression from mania to utter depression in manic-depressive disease. As this disease develops, the periods of stimulation become increasingly shorter and less frequent, while the periods of withdrawal, or depression, become longer and more common.

An unrecognized variation of exposure to an addicting substance may result in an unexpected increase in symptoms. A chronically tired beer drinker who is allergic to the grain in his brew may experience a sudden lift from a few shots of whisky (++) and then experience a delayed hangover (———), before returning to his accustomed state of fatigue (——).

A person with "brain-fag" (———), who is actually allergic to the cane sugar in his coffee, may experience a psychotic episode (++++) after eating a hot fudge sundae, loaded with such sugar. This may be followed by a deep depression, with an eventual return to his ordinary state of mental exhaustion. This hot-fudge-sundae side trip, superimposed on a long-standing susceptibility to cane sugar, might be represented by the following progression: minus-three, plus-four, and minus-four before a return to minus-three. All of this typically takes place without the victim himself understanding the source of the problem.

The stimulated food or chemical addict can go along for years without seeking medical advice. He is oblivious to the source of his problem and may not even know that he has a problem. Alcoholics, for instance, are notorious for their ability to deceive themselves about the extent of their problem. Advanced food addicts are no less self-deceiving.

The increasingly frequent hangovers, or minus reactions, bring the addict to the doctor. This onset of negative symptoms, either localized or systemic, is regarded by one and all as the "onset of the present illness." Except for a minority of patients, most addicts of this type are improperly diagnosed and treated. Usually they are given synthetic drugs, such as antihistamines, pain relievers, or tranquilizers.

Because of the hidden nature of food and chemical allergies, the orthodox doctor usually does not diagnose the demonstrable cause of the illness. Despite the individual nature of the problem, he gives some mass-applicable remedy and does not deal with the specific needs of the patient. And because of the polysymptomatic nature of the illness, he often dismisses the patient's many and varied complaints as signs of hysteria, neurosis, or hypochondria.

The result is that ecologic disturbances—which may be America's greatest single health problem—are often bypassed by the medical profession and only faintly glimpsed by its victims. Millions of people are undergoing needless drugging, hospitalization, or even surgery, because the environmental cause of their problem is not understood.

Adaptation

I have attempted to explain the concepts of clinical ecology in terms of adaptation to environmental exposures—a framework borrowed from physiology. In biology, when an organism comes into contact with a new element in its environment, it often responds in three stages: first, there tends to be an immediate acute reaction; this may be followed by an adapted stage in which there is a suppression of reactive symptoms; and finally, the organism may become maladapted, and perhaps later, nonadapted to repeated exposures by again presenting immediate, acute symptom responses.

Since new patients usually first come to their physicians midway in this process, they tend to present quite a different clinical picture than observed in laboratory animals. Instead of the sequence noted above, patients are first seen by their physicians as their adaptation to that to which they are susceptible is petering out. To what and for how long they had been adapted to such a frequently repeated exposure, which had maintained a relatively stimulatory phase, remain unknowns. Indeed, such a substance often appears to agree with an adapting person very well. But sooner or later—largely depending on the degree of individual susceptibility—such a person slips into a withdrawal phase for longer and longer periods. In other words, he completes this transition (usually called the onset of the present illness) and is now maladapted (badly adapted).

Such a transition from an adapted and relatively symptom-free existence to chronic illness often involves many side trips, including various levels. The speed with which this transition takes place is also partially dependent on the patient's awareness of his problem. If he remains totally unaware of the environmental cause(s) of his symptoms, the transition may take place fairly rapidly. If he is aware that eating in general, for instance, agrees with him, he may be able to slow the onset of maladaptation, although he may become progressively obese in the process. And finally, if the patient is aware of the particular food(s) related to his symptoms, he may be able to delay his ultimate downfall by a judicious intake of the particular culprit. Eventually, however, most patients lose their symptom-suppressed adaptation to such substances and wind up in a doctor's waiting room. Unfortunately, there is another outcome which may occur at any stage of this adaptation process to food(s). Some patients, suspecting that all food and/or food additives and contaminants make them ill, simply stop eating. This may lead to a marked loss of weight and hazardous undernutrition.

For the reader interested in greater detail, adaptation is defined as the ability of an organism to be modified in its function by the impingement of its environment. In the specific and individualized sense employed here, adaptation is limited to observed clinical manifestations resulting from the impingement of given environmental exposures to which individuals are highly susceptible.[2,3] Adolph also observed similar effects in animals.[4]

Environmental features contributing to specific adaptation are the following: a) Given exposures must be cumulative and preferably intermittent. Those substances, such as common foods, retained in the body temporarily are most effective in inducing and maintaining specific adaptation. b) Specific reexposures should be approximately the same size, and rate of absorption through a common portal of entry. c) Given environmental exposures may be harmless (foods) or alleged to be toxic in greater concentrations, although thought to be safe in the lesser amounts encountered (chemicals).

Bodily features contributing to specific adaptation include: ability of an individual to adapt; this probably depends on: a) inherited tendencies, b) adequacy of apparent physiologic mechanisms,[5-8] and c) variations in the degree of specific susceptibility, inasmuch as a heightened susceptibility seems to enhance the impact of lesser dosage and accelerates the advancement of the adaptation process.

Because of these environmental and bodily (individual) variants, adaptation to given environmental exposures develops and advances more rapidly in some individuals than in others. For instance, one person may present only a few localized syndromes from only a few environmental exposures, whereas another person may manifest many apparently different physical and more advanced cerebral and behavioral syndromes from multiple exogenous exposures. Moreover, such lesser and advanced responses may alternate in a given person at different times.[9] This alternation of what later were called allergies (rhinitis, asthma, eczema, and headache) with psychoses was apparently first pointed out in 1884 by George Savage, an English psychiatrist.[10]

In contrast to this highly individualized interpretation of adaptation to specific environmental exposures, traditionally physiological adaptation has been presented elsewhere in respect to its general features and common bodily mechanisms.[5-7] Since a given individual is adapting not only to common foods and lesser chemical exposures, but also to many other environmental stimuli—such as infection, cold, heat, radiation, etc.—the ability to adapt or maladapt must also be considered in a broader context. For instance, it is known that virus infections frequently induce or precipitate maladapted allergic responses to other materials. The same relationship holds for systemic yeast infections,[11] and sometimes other infectious processes. Adequate treatment of a concomitant infection in the management of allergies must always be considered. It is also well known that sudden exposure to cold in some persons may be generally deleterious. Although the relationship of these secondary factors in adaptation is important, a detailed discussion of them is beyond the scope of this popular presentation.

3
The Problem of
Chemical Susceptibility

The same sort of problems which are caused by hidden food allergies can also be caused by exposure to common environmental chemicals. Many people now know that such chemicals may have long-term, harmful effects on the body and may cause cancer and other diseases. The damage done actually goes far beyond this, however. Common environmental chemicals have become a major source of chronic illnesses of many types in the United States and other industrialized countries.

Knowledge of this problem emerged slowly from the study of food allergy. Dr. Albert Rowe, one of the fathers of this field, reported in the 1930s on a peculiar reaction which he called "multiple fruit sensitivity." A characteristic of this problem was that certain patients tended to become ill when they ingested a wide variety of fruits.

Susceptibility to fruit is fairly common, but usually such allergies center on one or more of the botanically distinct fruit families (see Appendix A). These patients, however, had allergies to most, or all, domestically grown fruit, including examples of up to ten different food families. It would be understandable for a person who was allergic to peaches also to be allergic to apricots, for they both form part of the same botanical group—the rose family. But why should a person react to peaches and also to, say, pineapples, bananas, and dates, which are members of two other distinctly different biological families?

I confirmed Rowe's observations in my own practice, but neither he nor I could offer any logical explanation of the problem, and our reports caused a good deal of scepticism among some of our colleagues.

CASE STUDY: HEADACHES

In the mid-1950s, William Petersen came to me as a patient, complaining that eating a single commercial apple would cause him to have a severe headache. Petersen was fed on apples twice in my office after having avoided this food for a week, and on both occasions was struck with searing attacks of head pain. I naturally diagnosed him as allergic to apples.

Petersen was an inquisitive man, with a determination to understand *why* he reacted in the way he did. He lived in a nearby state which had a large fruit-producing belt. Upon returning home, working on a hunch, he slipped into an abandoned orchard and gathered some apples from the trees. These apples had not been sprayed or cared for in years. He picked about half a peck of sound ones and took them home. Surprisingly, he was able to eat these unsprayed, untreated apples with complete abandon: he ate three or four of them at a time, every day for a week. He had no headache or any other reaction whatsoever. He then reported the result of his experiment to me.

I therefore obtained my own source of unsprayed apples and tested Petersen on these in my office. Again, he had no reaction to unsprayed apples but responded with a severe headache to any commercial variety. Petersen went on to eat apples thereafter, provided he obtained them from uncontaminated sources. He didn't have an apple allergy at all; he had something else, something which still did not have a name.

To extend this observation, in 1953 I obtained samples of apples sprayed with several major pesticides from the horticulture department of the College of Agriculture of the University of Illinois. By using these apples, as well as completely unsprayed and untreated ones, the problem of the "multiple fruit sensitivity" was finally worked out. The majority of the patients who reacted to these fruits were usually not allergic to fruit at all. What they were susceptibile to was the chemical pollution of fruit. The unsprayed fruit could be tolerated quite well, but the commercially available varieties, such as are obtained in supermarkets and fruit stores, caused chronic health problems such as arthritis, colitis, nervousness, and depression.

This observation raised a host of questions about health and sickness, questions which struck at the basis of much of Western technology.

How safe is our present chemical environment? To what extent does it contribute to chronic illness? How much do we know about the long-term effects of such by-products of "progress" as the chemical pollutants in the air of our homes and cities, chemical additives and contaminants in our foods, water, cosmetics, and drugs?

Supposedly these environmental chemicals had been tested and found safe.

However, there were serious questions to be asked about the validity of long-term toxicity studies carried out by government or industry. If only a minority of rats responded adversely to a chemical, were these results averaged out in the final report? What about the minority of people who are similarly afflicted? Were they being similarly ignored or lost in our statistical studies? These were important questions, since even if only one or two percent of the population were made chronically ill by daily exposure to such chemicals, this would still amount to two to four million people in the United States alone, enough to keep all our physicians busy for a long time. We doctors were the ones who had to deal with the unusual reactions, yet the medical profession seemed completely unaware of the potential danger.

Many of the chemicals in common use had become "profitable ventures" by the time anyone began to suspect that they were harmful. They thus became the focal point, individually and collectively, of defensive public relations operations by giant companies.

Indeed, some of the most troublesome chemical exposures have not been adequately described, and there is still no general knowledge of their potential hazards. The chief reason for this is that these materials have become integral parts of our current existence. Since they are so common, they are not usually suspected. Not being suspected, they are not usually avoided deliberately. Thus, not being eliminated either by chance or design, certain common chemical exposures remain unsuspected causes of chronic physical and "mental" illnesses.

There is an element of addiction to some of these chemicals, as well. Even though certain chemical exposures may be suspected of causing harm, avoidance is not only inconvenient, and sometimes expensive, but, because of the addictionlike responses that may be involved, sometimes the victims do not even wish to avoid exposure to the chemicals. Thus, understanding of this problem has been obstructed both by the constant nature of the chemical exposure and the self-perpetuation of the process.

I called this the chemical *susceptibility* problem, instead of the chemical *allergy* or *sensitivity* problem, to avoid prolonged and pointless debates over whether such small doses could cause classic allergic reactions. Whatever their name, such reactions were real and increasingly common, as many cases were to show.[1]

CASE STUDY: CHEMICAL SUSCEPTIBILITY

Nora Barnes came to me as a patient in 1947. Mrs. Barnes had been repeatedly diagnosed as a hypochondriac. No physician had been able to find the cause of her multiple symptoms and complaints.

In childhood she had been the victim of widespread allergies and had frequent problems with runny nose, cold sores, and outbreaks of hives. These went away as she grew to adulthood but were soon replaced by fierce headaches—blinding pain which sent her running to her bed. She suffered from persistent fatigue, irritability, nervousness, and tension. She also had a cough, which eventually turned into bronchial asthma.

At one time she had been employed as a cosmetics saleswoman. She noticed after a while that when she applied nail polish, her eyes would itch furiously. She soon had bags under her eyes, and the skin around them became red and inflamed. She applied make-up to hide this problem.

By the time she came to see me, she was in a wretched condition. She had had to drive through the industrial belt of northern Indiana to reach my office, and as she approached the city limits of Chicago, she felt sicker than ever. In the city, she practically caused an accident when she swung out of traffic to escape from the exhaust fumes of a bus.

Arriving at a hotel in Chicago's downtown Loop district, she was practically incoherent when she called me on the telephone. By chance, the desk clerk gave her a room on the twenty-third floor. Soon she felt somewhat better and attempted to go downstairs and do some shopping. But she found that when she went into the lobby or onto any floor below the twentieth, her nausea, dizziness, and feelings of suffocation returned.

She had had three experiences in which she had collapsed in a "drunken" stupor while driving her car. Only the fact that someone was in the passenger seat beside her prevented a serious accident. She often became ill while riding in the back seats of cars, but rarely in the front. Some cars, especially those with noisy mufflers, seemed worse than others.

All of this was confusing, but the single most intriguing fact in her case was that her symptoms became progressively worse after July Fourth and did not get any better until after Christmas. Between New Year's and Independence Day, she remained tolerably well, only to get miserably sick and "neurotic" again after the Fourth of July.

One possible explanation of this could be hay fever, but there were no pollens in her state which were troublesome during that particular period. In the course of our conversation, however, Nora mentioned that she always went to a cabin in the woods for the summer—on July Fourth. Something in that cabin, I felt, might be responsible for these various symptoms. By testing samples from her home, it turned out the main culprit was the pine paneling of the cabin. Pine was also burned in the fireplace, and various pine scented materials were used in the house, including disinfectants. When all pine products were removed from the cabin her symptoms improved.

Some time later, however, she and her husband went to a hunting lodge which had been heated by a fuel-oil stove. She began to cough and wheeze within a few minutes after entering the building, and became unconscious.

She reported that the odor of her gas kitchen range made her feel sick, as did those of her gas-burning home utilities, sponge rubber padding, plastic upholstered furniture, rubber mattress and pillow, and beds whose mattresses were encased in plastic coverings. She was able to effect real improvement by simply removing all these items from her home and replacing them with less offensive substitutes. Her Christmas-time malaise was traced to the pine Christmas tree.

The overall picture of Nora Barnes' illness did not strike home until one blustery day, when a fierce storm threatened the Chicago area. All other patients had cancelled their appointments, but Mrs. Barnes came in, and together we reviewed over fifty typewritten pages of her record. Finally, a pattern emerged. Almost all her problems could be traced back to petrochemicals, combustion products, or man-made chemicals manufactured from petroleum. Nora Barnes was allergic or susceptible to a wide range of supposedly safe environmental agents. Her susceptibility to pine and pine products fit into this picture, too, since our current supply of hydrocarbon fuels is believed to be derived, ultimately, from a huge prehistoric pine forest, crushed beneath the earth.

This theory led to new revelations in Mrs. Barnes' case. By eliminating all plastics and chemicals from her life, she discovered that she could dramatically improve her health. Food stored in glass, for instance, could be eaten, but the same food stored in plastic containers made her sick.

A drink of creme de menthe invariably made her sick—in fact, she passed out on several occasions when trying to drink it. She now found out why: she was incredibly sensitive to all artificial food colorings and so she avoided not only this green liqueur, but also maraschino cherries, mint sauce, frankfurters, and similar products (see list, Chapter 4).

She noticed that canned tomatoes made her sick, but that she was able to eat tomatoes from her own garden. The problem was traced to the lining of the tin cans in which the commercial food was packed. Also, foods sprayed with insecticide would bring on headaches, whereas unsprayed food would not. She found that she could eat beef raised on a neighbor's farm but not commercially raised beef, which had been fed pesticide-treated feeds and sprayed for fly control.

The case of Nora Barnes provided a new perspective on medical practice. It soon became apparent that she was not alone, that many of the patients seen by physicians with similarly peculiar and multiple symptoms were actually suffering from allergies to synthetic chemicals. These people were not born this way. They acquired a high susceptibility because of constant, day-in and day-out exposure to chemicals, especially in the period since World War Two.

Almost inevitably, their susceptibility to chemicals intermingled with food allergies, to form an overall picture of environmental illness. These patients were reacting to foreign substances which are known to be toxic (poisonous). But it had always been assumed that reactions of toxicity occurred at much higher levels of exposure. These "chemical patients" reacted to minute amounts of contamination, which doctors until then had not considered problematic.

The full clinical implications of the chemical susceptibility problem developed over a number of years. As this environmentally oriented medical problem emerged, each new patient revealed some aspect or feature of this condition not previously appreciated. Full realization of the two most important sources of chemical pollution of the environment, namely, the contribution of gas utilities to indoor air pollution and the crucial roles of pesticide exposures in both indoor and outdoor (ambient) air pollution, did not become clear until Ellen Sanders came to me as a patient in early 1953.

CASE STUDY: CHEMICAL SUSCEPTIBILITY

Mrs. Sanders was a forty-four-year-old housewife and former personnel worker. For the previous seven years she had practically been a physical invalid. Since a child she had always suffered from headaches, backaches, stuffy nose, car sickness, and hyperactivity. Her various problems always seemed to get worse in the gas-equipped kitchen of her home. For instance, if she were asked to set the table, she would commonly drop a dish on the way from the kitchen cupboard to the dining room. This would usually trigger an emotional scene in her family. She never learned to cook as a child because of clumsiness, irritability, and crying when in the kitchen. Instinctively, she avoided the house, especially the kitchen, preferring to stay outdoors where, she said, there was "more air." Her face was commonly red. At school she was often accused of wearing rouge.

When she grew up and married, her problems increased. There was a marked intensification of all symptoms in the fall of 1947 when she painted a large apartment, having used paint and varnish removers freely in addition to being exposed to paint odors over a two-week period. Thereafter interminable colds, nasal stuffiness, and intermittent bouts of bronchitis were attributed to an unknown virus. She became acutely ill each time that she attempted to eat cherries and certain other fruits. Since she enjoyed pottery, she enrolled in a pottery class which was held in a poorly ventilated large room which also contained a gas-fired kiln and which was contaminated by fumes from painting, silk screening, and other art work. These exposures brought on attacks of asthma and were discontinued after two weeks. In the late 1940s she suffered constant attacks of "influenza," headache, nausea, and vomiting. She found that she could feel better by not eating at all and staying outdoors as much as possible. She lost 25 pounds in a single month and weighed only 85 pounds at one time.

Various doctors prescribed one medication after another, but each seemed to make her more sick than the last one. The top of her dresser came to resemble a pharmacist's counter. She took to drying her hair by the heat of her gas-fired oven, which helped to clear her asthma temporarily but was inevitably followed by severe headache, fatigue, depression, and, sometimes, loss of consciousness. Immediately prior to such acute episodes, her cheeks would turn fiery red, she would stagger around the room, bumping into the furniture. She was living in Arizona by this time, a state to which she had moved on the advice of her physicians. Initially, she felt much better, as long as she remained outdoors. But she was always worse on rainy days; this was attributed to the lack of exposure to Arizona sunshine, instead of to exposures when in her home. With the onset of colder weather in the fall, she became increasingly asthmatic, hyperactive, and confused with episodes of extreme hyperactivity and loss of consciousness.

Because of this strange behavior, her husband and doctor concluded that Mrs. Sanders was a drug addict, and that heroin or some such narcotic was responsible for her behavior. Her husband went so far as to beat her, trying to extract from this terrified woman the location of her "stash." This interpretation was supported by the fact that she improved when taken to a hospital, only to worsen immediately upon again returning to her home. Finally, her husband and her physician made plans to admit her to a mental institution.

Mrs. Sanders' brother was a physician who suspected that her illness might be in some way allergy-related. He brought her to me for treatment immediately before she was scheduled to be institutionalized. Upon entering an apartment the first night in Chicago, her brother lighted the gas range to prepare dinner. She immediately complained of the odor of gas, her face became red, her eyes crossed, and she was barely able to speak. Her brother called me in alarm, to explain what was happening to his sister. Suspecting some environmental exposure, I instructed him to remove her immediately. Fortunately, she was taken to a friend's all-electric apartment. By this time, her head was drawn to one side in a wry neck reaction (acute torticollis), she was confused, disoriented, and slumped into a semi-conscious stupor. This was interrupted by periods of uncontrollable twitching of muscles and flailing of all limbs so violently that she had to be physically restrained. She remained unconscious with intermittent seizures for the following six hours. In a similar attack a few months later, also followed by accidental exposure to gas, she was seen by a neurologist, who diagnosed her condition in these words: "Impression: cataleptic attack. I would strongly suspect hysteria."

Extensive testing, however, revealed that Ellen Sanders, like Nora Barnes, was highly susceptible to chemical environmental exposures. In particular, she was exquisitely sensitive to utility gas exposures. In retrospect, many of her previous problems, from the time that she dropped plates as a child to her most recent attacks, could be traced to gas exposures. However, she was also highly susceptible to many other environmental chemicals, especially pesticide sprays on foods, aerial spraying for mosquito abatement, automotive exhausts, and many others. Next to the effects of utility gas, pesticide exposures were the most troublesome. As little as half a commercially sprayed peach would induce "drunkenness," followed by loss of consciousness. But if she ate only so-called "organic" food and avoided chemical exposures, she remained well. Occasionally, however, during the past 25 years she has had accidentally induced acute reactions of the type described. Upon one occasion, she was accidentally exposed to pesticides when the outside of her apartment was sprayed to control an infestation of spiders. Within minutes after these fumes entered her apartment through an air conditioner, she again lapsed into unconsciousness temporarily. Severe chest pain persisted for several weeks before subsiding. This has happened on a few other occasions, although electrocardiograms, even after exercise, failed to show any abnormalities. More recently, both exposures to airborne pesticides and automotive exhausts have precipitated bouts of heart irregularity persisting for several hours. Other than for these intermittent exposures, she remains in good general health while following her environmentally restricted medical program.

These two cases opened up the field of chemical susceptibility. Although they are extreme instances, they are hardly unique. An increasing percentage of my patients have this chemical susceptibility problem to varying degrees. Some are aware that they cannot tolerate synthetic substances or combustion products. Others are sick, but do not yet realize why.

To recognize this problem is not to oppose progress. But we must distinguish between what is merely new and what is truly progressive. Since the mid-nineteenth century chemistry has revolutionized modern life. The United States alone produces over 500 billion pounds of chemicals per year. There are now about four million chemicals in the computer register of the Chemical Abstract Service. About 33,000 of these are in common use in the United States,[2] and many of these ultimately find their way into our bodies. What are the health effects of these chemicals individually or, more importantly, cumulatively? Despite the Toxic Substances Control Act of 1976, very few of these chemicals have been adequately tested before being introduced into the marketplace.

In the last thirty years copious evidence has accumulated that these chemicals can indeed cause serious health problems for workers and consumers. There are many Nora Barnses and Ellen Sanderses walking around or dragging themselves from one doctor's office to another.

As with the case of food, a constructive criticism of the chemical industry is sometimes taken as a threat to profit and unreasonably opposed. At the present time, the chemical companies are spending many millions of dollars to convince the public that their products are safe and indispensable. This money would be better spent investigating the actual damage that uncontrolled chemical contamination does and in devising ways to control it.

Formaldehyde

As with certain other chemical exposures, inhalation of formaldehyde odors also causes severe allergic symptoms in susceptible persons, although it has long been associated with apparent toxicity. Dr. David L. Morris of LaCrosse, Wisconsin, is responsible for calling this problem to the attention of clinicians.

According to Dr. Morris, formaldehyde is manufactured from low molecular weight petroleum products and is usually sold as formalin. Formalin is used extensively in industry as a disinfectant and in making urea resins and other plastics. Odors of formaldehyde are found in fabric and new clothing stores. Formaldehyde resins are used widely in making plywood, paneling and particle board, as well as in permapress and wash-and-wear fabrics. In recent years, formaldehyde preparations have been used extensively in the manufacture of latex paint, mobile homes, and, especially, in home insulating materials.

Exposure to formaldehyde can cause all the recognized symptoms of inhalant and contact allergy. These include respiratory, skin, and gastrointestinal symptoms. More advanced reactions include fatigue, headache, muscle and joint aches and pains, and cerebral symptoms.

4

The Chemicals in Our Food

We have spoken of the problems of food allergy and chemical susceptibility as the two main components of environmental disease. This is technically correct, but in actuality these two problems are usually found together, tightly interlinked in the history of each chronically ill individual. One of the major ways in which these two elements interlock is in the chemical pollution of our food supply.

It is no secret that our food is now treated with synthetic chemicals of every sort. Some of these chemicals have been deliberately added, to impart color, flavor, or longer shelf life. These deliberately added substances are called *additives*. In addition, numerous chemicals accidentally enter the food supply as residues of pesticides, fertilizers, or environmental pollutants. These are called food *contaminants*.

Together, food additives and food contaminants have become a major source of the problem of chemical susceptibility in most Western countries, since everyone must eat, and most food now comes from the giant agribusiness conglomerates. These giant corporations are mainly concerned with maximizing profit, even if the health consequences for the population are negative. What is more, these companies are often closely linked to chemical companies and thus have a built-in bias in favor of synthetic pesticides and fertilizers.[1]

For any person who wants to avoid environmentally induced illness, it is necessary to understand the sources of such chemical contamination of the food supply. These chemicals can either cause, or help perpetuate, chronic illnesses of all sorts. However, their presence can be detected, and they themselves can be avoided, by methods which are explained later in this book.

I have already described how the role of chemical pesticides was discovered in the case of William Petersen, the man who found that he could eat unsprayed apples from an abandoned orchard, while commercial apples from a store gave him a headache. The principles discovered in this case were soon extended to many other food-allergy patients. It was determined that in some cases they were actually reacting only to chemical contaminants. Usually, however, patients with the chemical susceptibility problem also had the food allergy problem, and vice versa.

Some patients appeared to react to commercial food in the winter, but to a much lesser degree in the warmer months. This was because in the cold months they were often cooped up in their houses and exposed to the cumulative effects of indoor air pollution (Chap. 6). The *combination* of food allergies, contaminated food, and such indoor pollutants greatly heightened their symptoms and made their winters miserable. Not infrequently their winter maladies, environmental in origin, masqueraded as colds or flus. In other cases, they did have genuine infections, but these were accentuated by allergic problems.

The variety of problems is endless, since environmental disease is above all things an *individual* problem. There is no single cause for all people, nor a single solution. Usually the disease is a result of the interaction between an individual, with his particular bodily makeup, and his environment. Certain exposures, however, stand out as most troublesome for the greatest number of patients. Of the food additives and contaminants, some of the most troublesome are residues of pesticide sprays which find their way into almost everything the average person eats.

Spray Residues

In order to further study the question of spray residues and their effect on health, I asked three of my patients to take part in an experiment. Each of them was known to be susceptible to a wide range of chemicals. I invited them to my office for a peach-eating session, using fruit from the local market. After eating these commercial peaches, one patient developed a rash, with itching, burning and stinging, and the formation of red wheals (urticaria). The second had a frightening attack of asthma. The third developed a headache. To make the test complete, similar-looking peaches were obtained from an abandoned orchard where the fruit grew wild, unblessed by the exterminator's spraygun.

After an interval, the three were given some of these peaches, without their being identified as unsprayed fruit. To these items they had no reaction at all: they tolerated them perfectly well. In the following season, I tested 15 more patients in a more elaborate experiment which was mentioned briefly in the previous chapter. I obtained four lots of peaches, all of the same type, but each treated quite differently. The first were picked from trees in an abandoned orchard, having received no sprays, fungicidal treatment, or fertilization for the previous three years. The second lot were the same as the first, except that they had been manually dusted with sulfur as an antifungus measure. The third were from one of the University of Illinois plots which had received the recommended spray schedules using DDT and dieldrin. The fourth were peaches from the same source sprayed with the pesticides parathione and dieldrin.

For several days before the test, all of the patients avoided both peaches and chemicals to which they knew they were susceptible. The patients were assembled in my office and were given the various peaches, without any knowledge of which batch they were receiving. Three of the fifteen became ill when they ate plain, uncontaminated peaches. They were evidently allergic to peaches per se. A larger number of the others reacted to both the sulfured and the sprayed peaches. Some of them became so ill, in fact, that they refused to go on with the testing. This was good common sense on their part, but it detracted from the completeness of the experiment. Nevertheless, several of those who had no reaction to the organic peaches were made ill by the sprayed peaches, regardless of the type of spray used. Clearly there were people who were made sick by eating infinitesimally small amounts of insect spray, similar to the amounts millions of people eat every day.

One good effect of this discovery was that patients who had long stopped eating fruit, from the belief that they were made sick by it, were able to start again, provided they ate only organically grown, uncontaminated fruits.

"Multiple fruit sensitivity" turned out to be not such a very rare condition. An investigation of spraying practices exposed some of the underlying reasons for this problem. Peaches, apples, and cherries were the most commonly contaminated, as well as the most heavily contaminated, fruits. Although the total number of spraying applications varied with rainfall and other conditions, peaches, apples, and cherries were often sprayed between ten and fifteen times each season. Recommended spraying started with blossoming and ended only a few weeks prior to harvesting. Needless to say, these fruit were fairly well saturated with spray.

They are hardly unique in this respect, however. It turned out that most of the commercially produced fruits in the United States are *copiously sprayed*. Some of them are sprayed with many different agents, and it became almost an impossible task to decide which spray caused which symptom in a patient. This problem has increased year by year.

Once a fruit has been sprayed with a combination of pesticide and kerosene, or some other chemical solvent, *there is no known way of removing the spray residue*. Air passes quite readily through the skin of a piece of fruit and with it comes the spray ingredients, to be incorporated into the pulp itself. Washing, rubbing, peeling, cooking, and any other attempt to clean the spray off do not eliminate spray residues. The experimental proof of this assertion is the chemically sensitive patient, who gets sick from commercial, sprayed fruit no matter how he rubs or washes it.

Some individuals, however, who are not violently susceptible to chemicals, may be able to eat stewed fruit, but not raw, fresh specimens of the same lot. The reason appears to be that when the fruit is stewed, some of the pesticides are boiled off. Some of my patients have, in fact, gotten sick simply by standing over a pot of stewing commercial fruit, inhaling the vapors which contain part of the pesticides escaping into the atmosphere. Stewing organically grown fruit does not have that effect on these patients, however.

It must be emphasized that a highly susceptible person, eating an ordinary diet, rarely suspects the fact that a daily piece of fruit causes any problem at all. The reason for this is that the small, daily dose of pesticide may merely serve to reinforce and perpetuate his symptoms of illness. All he knows is that he felt badly yesterday and feels just as badly today. He naturally does not associate his headache or his asthma or his fatigue with something so innocent, and apparently unconnected, as the supposedly beneficial fruits and vegetables. It is only when he overindulges and takes in an extraordinary amount of these products (and pesticide) that he breaks out of the level of chronic disease and precipitates an obvious reaction.

Multiple Vegetable Sensitivity

People who are sensitive, or susceptible, to chemicals are often unable to eat cabbage, broccoli, cauliflower, celery, lettuce, spinach, beet greens, and certain other leafy vegetables. Often such people will simply think such vegetables "do not agree with them." This may be the case—that is, they *may* be suffering from allergies to one or more of these foods.

Some patients, however, are susceptible to the effects of *sprayed* vegetables but not to the same vegetables when they are unsprayed. The worst culprits in this respect seem to be the various members of the cabbage family (including cabbage, broccoli, and cauliflower). They are among the most heavily contaminated vegetables. One sign of this may be that until about 1950, all cooks were warned to look out for cabbage worms on broccoli. Since that time, however, no one of my acquaintance has found one of these insects on commercial broccoli. This certainly represents progress for the cook—but progress at what price?

Another practice which has contributed to the contamination of foods is the indiscriminate spraying of fruit and vegetable counters in stores and supermarkets. This is done to control bugs, molds, and especially flies, which can be unsanitary. The almost complete absence of fruit flies, even in summer, is a testimony to the effectiveness of this spraying program. Susceptible persons, however, may start to cough, wheeze, or show other signs of a reaction when they enter the fruit and vegetable section of a store. Often, of course, this reaction cannot be distinguished from a reaction to the many other chemicals one is likely to encounter in a supermarket.

The Chemical Contamination of Meat

Meat also may be contaminated by sprays, especially the fat of lamb, beef, and some poultry. The main culprit here appears to be the chlorinated hydrocarbons, which enter the animals' bodies by way of *sprayed feed*. In addition, on many ranches the animals themselves are routinely sprayed to control flies and other insects.

In most cases, reactions to meat can be greatly reduced by cutting off all fat prior to cooking. Nevertheless, some individuals who are very susceptible to chemicals still react badly to beef or lamb which has had most of the fat removed. These same individuals, however, generally do not react to uncontaminated meat.

Fumigant Contamination

Federal law dictates that dates and many other dried fruits must be fumigated with a chemical called methyl bromide before they are shipped across state lines. Thus, almost all of the dates eaten in this country contain a small but often troublesome residue of this chemical.

Many people have noticed that dates and figs are laxatives and even eat them for this purpose. However, in my experience, it is not mainly the fruit itself which exerts this laxative effect but the chemical contamination. *Unsprayed* figs or dates can usually be eaten with impunity, even in one- or two-pound lots, *without* causing any laxative action at all. An exception would be a person who is allergic, or sensitive, to dates or figs per se and reacts by getting an upset stomach.

The same problem can be observed with nuts, dried peas, beans, and lentils, all of which are heavily fumigated. Many people believe that they simply cannot eat these foods without having a reaction, but when they try "organic" varieties of the same foods, or nuts *in the shell*, they do not have the reactions.

Health-conscious people often try to protect themselves by buying *unsulfured* dried fruit. Such apricots, pears, peaches, and so forth may indeed be unsulfured, but they are generally not uncontaminated. Most of the so-called "health food" dried fruit has been sprayed and fumigated and will often cause the same problems for chemically susceptible people as the commercial variety.

In the early 1960s, I conducted a test among my patients to determine the possible effects of chemical contamination of wheat and corn—the two leading causes of food allergy. Both foods were avoided for five days prior to the test feedings. Patients were then given commercially available wheat and corn, and reactions to these were compared to those to cereal grains from a farm on which no commercial fertilizers and sprays had been used for thirty years. Although the frequency of food allergy to wheat and corn is approximately the same, more persons reacted to commercial corn products than to commercial wheat products. This difference may have been due to the fact that corn is often soaked in sulfur dioxide for several days in order to separate different parts of the kernel. Most manufactured corn products start from such chemically contaminated sources.

A similar problem is posed by bleaching agents used to whiten flour. It is difficult to separate the contribution of the bleach in white bread from the host of other chemicals which go into the loaf.

Sulfur

It is similarly not easy to separate the effects of sulfur from that of the many other contaminants and chemicals in our food. What is certain is that *sulfur is a major chemical contaminant* of our food supply.

Sulfur can bring on acute mental and physical symptoms. One woman, in a food test with peaches, did not react to uncontaminated peaches. But when she ate peaches which had been dusted with sulfur, within twenty minutes she began complaining of nervousness and tenseness. She began sweating profusely, only to get the chills moments later. After half an hour, she reported feeling nauseated. Five minutes later she vomited. Forty minutes after the test began she remained cold, her skin was clammy, and she was pale and depressed. Although her stomach was pumped, she continued to have severe stomach cramps, aches, fatigue, and depression for the rest of the day.

Some patients have wondered why they are unable to eat French fried potatoes in restaurants but can eat them at home with no trouble. The answer is that almost all restaurants buy preprocessed French fries which have been dipped in a solution of sulfur dioxide to stop them from browning. The same sulfur treatment is often given to potato chips and even to freshly cut apples and peaches in restaurants.

It is even more surprising to learn that some fresh produce, notably asparagus, is pretreated with a solution of sulfur dioxide to give it a more "attractive" color.

The processing of corn begins with the soaking of the whole kernel in a sulfur dioxide solution. This practice avoids fermentation of the corn while it is being processed but also seems to impart sulfur contamination to all manufactured corn products. This includes corn meal, cornstarch, corn flour, corn syrup, corn sugar, and corn oil.

Artificial Colors

Artificial colors have received a great deal of attention in recent years. Some of them have been removed from the marketplace by the Food and Drug Administration. Most recently, Red Dye No. 2 was removed after tests showed that it caused cancer in experimental animals.[2]

Long before this, however, starting in the late 1940s, clinical ecologists such as Dr. Stephen D. Lockey warned that artificial colors in drugs were one of the major sources of health problems in adults and children.[3]

To prove this, I once asked three chemically susceptible patients to take part in an experiment. They were blindfolded and given a glass of spring water to drink. Into each glass had been added the same amount of Red Dye No. 2 that would be found in a large serving of a well-known gelatin dessert. (This was before the link between the dye and cancer had been established.) Two of the three developed severe reactions to this colored water, although they had no reaction to pure spring water.

The practice of coloring fresh foods can also be a source of problems. Oranges, in particular, are frequently dyed, on the theory that consumers will not purchase naturally colored oranges, which are occasionally specked with green. It is difficult to detect a reaction to this dye, because fresh citrus fruits are often packed in crates which have been liberally treated with fungicides, and thus it is difficult to tell if the reaction is to the dye or to the fungicide.

Sweet potatoes are also commonly dyed. But dyed sweet potatoes can usually be eaten if they are carefully peeled. As a practical note, you can generally spot a dyed sweet potato by noting the presence of the dye on the broken ends of the tubers. Increasingly, in recent years, food wholesalers have begun dyeing white potatoes red. A list of other commercially colored foods follows.

FOODS THAT ARE COMMONLY DYED WITH ARTIFICIAL COLORS
Creme de menthe
Maraschino cherries and other colored fruit
Jello and other colored gelatin desserts
Mint sauce
Colored ice cream—unless label states otherwise
Colored sherbet
Colored candy

Cookie and pie frostings and fillings
Wieners
Bologna
Cheese
Butter
Oleomargarine
Oranges
Sweet potato
Irish potato
Root beer
Soda pop
Cola drinks and certain other soft drinks

CASE STUDY: EPILEPTICLIKE SEIZURES

Jim Garry was a typical American teenager; he was an average student, who enjoyed sports and was beginning to take an interest in girls. His diet, however, left much to be desired. He would fill up on snacks and down endless glasses of an artificially flavored and colored grape drink. Over a period of more than a year, Jim's strength began to fail him, and he showed less and less interest in his work or his friends. Then, one day, the seizures began. His parents, alarmed, took Jim to a neurologist. The doctor suspected epilepsy, yet the electroencephalogram (EEG) was normal. When the seizures continued, a psychiatrist was recommended, but the parents, suspecting allergy, brought him to me.

Jim avoided all soft drinks, all sugar, and especially all products made from grapes for a week. We then reintroduced into his diet, one by one, chemically uncontaminated grapes, commercial grape juice, and various kinds of sugar. There was no reaction; in fact, he felt better than he had in months. Then he was given a big glass of the same "junk food" soft drink to which he had been addicted. Within minutes, he fell to the floor, his body stiffened, and he went into what looked like a typical epileptic seizure.

When he recovered, a few minutes later, I discussed the cause of these seizures and the fatigue with him and his mother. I explained that chemicals in the environment, and especially food, can be a cause of these symptoms, and that if Jimmy wanted to regain his strength and health, he would have to stay away from *all* contaminated foods and other major chemical exposures. As long as he did this, he was not troubled with these problems again.

Foods Exposed to Gas

Although we rarely think about it, many of the foods we eat have been exposed to natural or synthetic gas. Small but potentially harmful residues of this gas may remain in these foods and cause problems for susceptible individuals.

Most bananas, for instance, are artificially ripened by exposure to ethylene gas immediately before they are distributed to the markets. The more time that elapses after this gassing, the more readily the bananas are tolerated by those who are highly susceptible to chemical exposures. This is apparently why chemically susceptible people are sometimes able to eat bananas and sometimes are not. There is a fairly certain way, however, to detect gassed bananas. The naturally ripened bananas have black seeds and tend to have small, specked spots on their skins, in contrast to the gassed bananas, which have immature white seeds and large blackened areas of the skin at points where they were bruised in handling or shipping.

One of the most common forms of food allergy is suceptibility to coffee. Many people are made chronically ill from the steady and habitual drinking of this, our national "grown-up" drink. But when patients with alleged coffee allergies were given electrically roasted coffee in an office test, some of them had no reaction at all. They only reacted to coffee which had been roasted over a gas flame. Almost all commercial coffee is gas-roasted, however. How much this fact contributes to the high incidence of susceptibility to coffee has not been investigated adequately.

The difficulty of separating the effects of chemicals and foods is illustrated by the following episode. In 1950, I co-authored an article on apparent susceptibility to sugarcane in a medical journal.[4]

Six patients were each given a glass of spring water with two heaping teaspoons of cane sugar dissolved in it. Each of them showed some adverse reactions to the drink, ranging from dizziness to sudden, uncontrollable fatigue.

We published these findings, feeling quite certain that these patients were sensitive to cane sugar per se. As I learned more about the effects of chemical contaminants in food, however, I realized that these patients may have been reacting to something other than sugar itself.

I visited a large sugar refinery and observed the process by which sugar is converted from rough cane to fine, white crystals for the table. Suspicions of chemical contamination centered on one particular stage in this process, *clarification*, when the cane syrup is filtered through roasted animal bones (called "bone char"). From time to time, these filters are washed, dried, and then reactivated at 1,000°F. over a gas-fired flame. It is highly likely that the char absorbs some of the combustion products of the gas. The sugar then picks up microscopic particles of this gas: not enough to taste or see, but enough to trigger a reaction by chemically susceptible patients.

In order to check this idea, several patients with *other* aspects of the chemical problem, who appeared to be also susceptible to cane, were tested with a special lot of cane sugar. This lot had been manufactured by means of a process which bypassed the bone-char filter. The test was "blind," in that the patients did not know whether they were receiving the special or the normal commercial sugar. Several of the patients became sick from the uncontaminated sugar; they were truly susceptible to cane. But a surprising number of those who had believed themselves unable to eat sugar discovered, to their surprise, that they could eat the unfiltered sugar with impunity. (Beet and corn sugar are also manufactured by similar processes.)

Containers

So many plastics and other materials are used today to pack food that it is difficult to sort out their contribution to the problem of chemical susceptibility. There is no doubt, however, that the packaging material, in its cumulative effect, is a major source of contamination for chemically susceptible people.

For example, some people are made ill by food stored in covered plastic freezer dishes, while eating some of the same lot of food before it is stored causes no problem. A few highly susceptible people will even react to foods stored in open glass containers in *plastic-lined* refrigerators. These same individuals can tolerate food which is stored in tightly fitted glass dishes so long as it is not exposed to the air in the plastic refrigerator. Fortunately for such patients, ecologically better enamel-lined refrigerators are being manufactured once again, after a lapse of several years.

As a rule of thumb, the more you can smell or bend a plastic, the more apt it is to contaminate food. Also, the longer the food is stored in such a container, and the more liquid the food, the more likely it is that chemical contamination will occur.

CASE STUDY: FUNGICIDE SUSCEPTIBILITY

Have you ever noticed a peculiar, acrid odor in fruit and vegetable markets? This smell may very well be coming from the crates used to pack citrus fruits, which are impregnated with fungicide. This is a good way to stop the growth of molds on cartons but can cause serious health problems for those inhaling the vapors. One patient, Doris Meredith, carelessly took a peck of citrus fruit in a fungicide-impregnated case into her home. Every time she entered the part of her house where the cartons were stored, she couldn't seem to catch her breath and began to wheeze uncontrollably.

Her husband eventually suspected that spray residue on the oranges was the cause and therefore washed each orange in hot, soapy water, drying each fruit separately. The odor still lingered, however, and continued to cause Mrs. Meredith to have acute respiratory symptoms.

Somewhat later, when she and her husband were moving to a new home, she became acutely ill and was confined to her bed, complaining of asthma and headaches. Her husband then recalled that her asthma had started shortly after the packing cases (citrus boxes) were brought into the home. Her symptoms subsided after the boxes were removed but recurred when the same boxes were brought back into the house (this time without her knowledge).

This woman also became depressed for days whenever she ate commercially available oranges. Her depression was so severe that she had contemplated going to a psychiatrist. However, treatment by the methods of clinical ecology was more effective in locating the cause of her problem, namely, fungicide residues, and in eliminating future such instances. She found, for example, that she could eat organic oranges with impunity—that is, oranges which had not been sprayed, dyed, or packed in fungicide-treated cartons.

We are just now beginning to understand the full power of these chemicals. For example, we now know that packing cases and express cars which have been contaminated with insecticides retain this contamination for long periods of time and may subsequently contaminate other loads.

This type of "second-hand" contamination may explain why some people are made ill by wheat which is shipped in paper or cardboard containers for long distances but not from the same organic wheat when it is shipped in metal containers. Some of the pesticides in the railroad car or truck manages to seep into the grain which is packed in porous paper.

Although cases such as Mrs. Meredith's are extreme instances, the fact that they occur underlines the need for chemically susceptible patients to have local sources of supply, so that food can be transferred from producer to consumer without becoming contaminated.

A more common source of container problems is the ubiquitous "tin" can, now usually made of aluminum or steel. Certain patients react to canned foods, while tolerating the same foods raw or uncanned with no trouble. I had made this observation often enough but could not figure out a way to separate the contribution of the can and its golden-brown phenol lining from that of the various sprays and chemicals found in processed foods. Phenol-containing compounds are used on the inside of tin cans to prevent the metal from bleaching the color of the food. I was finally able to make this distinction when a relative who lived in the state of Washington sent me some salmon which she and her husband had caught and "put up" in glass jars, as well as some tomatoes which had also been home-grown and packed.

When these foods were given to selected patients, they had no reaction. But when these same patients were later given salmon and tomatoes from commercial cans, lined with the golden-brown coating, they all became sick.

These patients have been able to eat fresh or home-packaged salmon or tomatoes since then with no difficulty. It is only when they try to eat such food in cans with phenol lining that they run into trouble.

Admittedly, only a minute amount of the resins and other chemicals used to line cans gets into the food. Is this really enough to cause a reaction? Yes, it is! Think of the difference in *taste* between canned and uncanned salmon, peaches, or other foods. Some of the characteristic "canned" taste of these foods comes from the substances in the lining, which seep into the food itself. If you can taste it, it can certainly have an effect on your health as well.

Patients who have suffered from depression, asthma, headache, and other symptoms have found relief of their long-term problems by avoiding chemicals and also by eliminating canned foods from their diets.

Waxes

Although many shoppers are unaware of the fact, certain fruits and vegetables are sold with a coating of paraffin wax. The wax on parsnips and rutabagas is so thick that you can scrape it off with your fingernail. But other so-called fresh produce, such as cucumbers, green peppers, and apples, are often sprayed with a light coating of paraffin to improve their appearance and shelf life. Not surprisingly, this petroleum-derived wax can contribute to the health problems of susceptible persons.

Some people think it is safe to eat such foods if they simply peel the wax away. But wax particles stick to the cut surfaces of waxed fruits and vegetables. To prove this, you simply have to peel a parsnip or other heavily waxed vegetable and then dip it into boiling water. Wax droplets may rise to the surface of the water, despite the fact that you supposedly removed the wax through peeling.

Peeling a commercial cucumber or apple is more effective in removing the wax. But these produce may still contain other chemical residues that can cause problems.

Antibiotics and Hormones

Since the end of World War Two, a staggering array of synthetic hormones, tranquilizers, and antibiotics, has been used to treat meat, poultry, and fish.

The most common hormone used for this purpose—diethylstilbesterol, or DES—was given as a medicine to pregnant women to prevent miscarriage. It is now known that the substance has caused cancer in the children of women who used it, the so-called "DES babies." The United States government is now waging a major campaign to warn such children, the potential victims, of the danger that was incurred.

For years, however, this hormone and other related substances, such as

Ralgro and Zeranol, were implanted in chickens, cattle, and sheep to make them grow fatter and come to market sooner. Industry has argued that only minute amounts of the chemicals were left in the meat which reached the consumer. But a growing number of scientists countered that it only took a few *parts per billion* to cause cancer in experimental animals.[5]

In addition to the use of hormones, it is common practice to inject animals with tranquilizers just before they are slaughtered and to dip certain foods (such as fish) in an antibiotic solution, to prevent them from spoiling. One of my patients became sick from eating store-bought fish. One day, her husband went deep sea fishing and brought back some fresh bluefish. She had no adverse reaction to this fish and soon learned that she could eat most freshly caught fish with impunity. She could also eat pieces of large commercial fish which were sawed into small portions while still frozen. Her problem apparently arose from the *antibiotic solution* which the industry routinely uses to treat smaller fresh fillets.

Organic Foods

A great deal more needs to be learned about the health effects of chemicals in our food. Chemical preservatives added to food cause problems in some patients. So, too, do chemicals used in fertilizing the soil. Because of concern over the way food is grown, a fairly large organic, or health food movement has grown up in recent years. While in general this is a good development, the reader should be aware that many so-called organic farms employ insecticides or fumigants, some of which are even required by law. More than once I have had to advise my patients not to patronize a certain health-food store or "organic" farm because one of their products was obviously contaminated: it made chemically susceptible patients sick.

The current state of agriculture is highly unsatisfactory from the point of view of anyone concerned about the contamination of food by chemicals. Only those farms and stores can be considered truly organic whose products are well-tolerated by a large group of patients susceptible to multiple chemicals, no matter how scrupulously they may try to avoid the use of chemicals. Sometimes economic pressure has induced reliable farms to start using chemicals to insure against loss, improve the yield, or increase the keeping qualities of their produce. In the United States, the organic food movement is handicapped by the manner in which huge companies dominate the thinking at the major agricultural colleges and government agencies.

Because of the difficulty of producing really pure food, the person who needs chemically less-contaminated produce should be prepared to pay premium prices for it. As expensive as this may be, it is never as expensive as the endless, agonizing trips to the doctor, only to be told in one way or another that the problem is "all in your head."

The Water Supply

Water is something we all take in, every day. It is obvious that the quality of that water will have a bearing on health and well-being. To prevent the spread of infectious diseases, such as typhoid fever, our cities began adding the chemical *chlorine* to the drinking water in 1912.

Chlorine was admirably effective in stopping the spread of infection. But, as a historian of this topic notes, "In discovering that drinking water could be purified by different filters, and made doubly safe through chlorination, interest in pollution declined."[6] Thus, there was very little reaction when two allergists, S. H. Watson and C. S. Kibler, showed, in 1934, that chlorinated drinking water could cause asthma in certain susceptible individuals.[7]

Chlorine is, in fact, a *common* cause of symptoms in individuals who are generally susceptible to chemicals. For this reason, in my special diagnosis and treatment facility, the Ecology Unit (Chap. 17), patients are given spring water to drink and treat chlorinated tap water as a "suspect" beverage. Some patients also react to swimming in chlorinated pools or even breathing their vapors. Some people are made sick by standing over a tub of steaming water in a closed bathroom. The contribution of fluoridation to this problem has simply not been studied adequately to permit us to make any definite statements about it.

In some parts of the country, the water is very "hard" (that is, saturated with mineral salts) and difficult to use in washing. There is a tendency in these areas to soften all water entering the kitchen or the laundry room with chemical water softeners. This is one of the built-in hazards of present-day home construction. If the softened water is drunk, it is apparently tolerated by many but a minority may become highly susceptible and be made ill by it.

The solution is to use softened water for all other purposes, but only *unsoftened* water for drinking and cooking. This requires having an extra tap in the kitchen. Some patients have a separate tap of unsoftened and filtered water, which is the only kind they use for internal consumption.

Even a "safe" source of water can easily become polluted. Certain wells, known to have been approved for use by chemically susceptible persons at one time, have since become chemically contaminated, as judged by several patients with this type of problem who are no longer able to use waters from such sources. The same holds true for several recently diagnosed patients.

Ideally, drinking waters should be rotated in the same way as foods. Of the recently hospitalized patients whom we have tested, approximately 70 percent reacted to one or several of the seven different waters which we routinely employed in testing. As with foods, a currently tolerated water may eventually become the source of individual reactions at some later time, especially if it is abused. Unfortunately, water rotation often is not practicable, since many locations lack an adequate variety of water supplies.

It should be said in summary that, as with other aspects of the food and chemical susceptibility problem, no two patients are found to have exactly the same water problem. For instance, there is no readily available water which seems to agree with all chemically susceptible patients, and a water which is agreeable to one person may be a major cause of symptoms in another. In short, the water problem remains not only highly individualized, but is also a common cause of persistent unexplained symptoms in otherwise controlled patients.

5

The Dangers of Drugs, Cosmetics, and Perfumes

One of the most ironic features of the chemical-susceptibility problem is that it is often begun, or at least perpetuated, by doctors themselves. To a large degree it can be considered an iatrogenic illness, that is, one that is induced by medical treatment.

The vast majority of drugs are synthetic and almost all of these contain petrochemical derivatives. Not infrequently, a patient who is unknowingly susceptible to petrochemicals will go to a conventional doctor for treatment. Let us say that the patient's problem is headache, caused by exposure to natural gas, synthetic fibers, and fumes.

The doctor diagnoses the headache as being stress-related, and tells the patient to try to relax more. In addition, he prescribes a pain-killer containing aspirin and other synthetic substances. When the patient takes this pain-killer, however, he may aggravate his already existing susceptibility to chemicals. In other words, instead of getting better, in the long run his headache problem may become worse. In addition, now he begins to suffer from mental confusion. Because of the increasing chemical load, he has moved, at least temporarily, from a minus-two category to a minus-three.

And so he returns to the physician, complaining of fatigue and possibly depression or "brain-fag," as well as intensified headache. The physician, not seeing the root cause of the problem, prescribes stronger drugs and advises the patient to take a vacation or see a psychologist. The stronger drugs bring on other reactions and visits to other specialists, in a downward spiral of symptoms and misguided treatments. By this point, the effects of the original chemical exposures have become more burdensome, since chemicals react in a cumulative fashion.

The patient may suspect that the doctor's prescription pad is the cause of some of his reactions, but he rarely suspects the full extent of the chemical problem. Consequently, even a cessation of all medication is unlikely to bring complete relief. The patient muddles along, with temporary improvements and persistent relapses in a generally downward course. The result is usually a frustrated physician and a patient who has become a very bitter dropout from the conventional medical system.

This problem is especially serious because in recent years there has been an explosion in the use of drugs as medicines in industrialized countries. Sales of prescription drugs alone, at the wholesale level, total over $9 billion in the United States.[1] This figure is practically double what it was a decade ago. Some of these drugs, of course, have been highly useful, even lifesaving, but often they have been misused and overprescribed, especially to those who are susceptible to their effects.

It is generally well known that drugs can, and often do, have serious side effects. Usually, however, these well-publicized side effects are of the *acute* kind: they bring on an immediate and highly visible reaction. As with allergies to rarely eaten foods, allergies to uncommonly encountered drugs are fairly easy to detect. If a person with little exposure to penicillin develops an allergy to it, the physician who dispensed the medication can usually tell that a reaction is taking place. Treatment then consists in finding an acceptable substitute and avoiding penicillin.

Acute reactions to drugs, however, are only the tip of the iceberg. Often, a drug will initiate or complicate a general intolerance for synthetic chemicals in the patient. These reactions are difficult to detect, since they come on insidiously. Usually, neither the patient nor the physician connects the heightened symptoms with the drug. The effects of the drug merge into the general background of chemical exposures.

All drugs, no matter how innocent they seem, can have side effects. The reactions may be caused by the active agent in the drugs, but they also can be caused by hidden ingredients such as flavorings, colorings, preservatives, and excipients, which are binders used in the manufacturing process. Few people realize the complexity of most drugs or the number of ingredients they contain. The ingredients of pharmaceuticals are rarely given on the label. An investigation of one over-the-counter preparation of synthetic vitamins revealed the presence of dozens of chemicals. In addition to seventeen vitamins and minerals, the pills contained calcium stearate as a lubricant, gelatin, sugar, sodium benzoate (a preservative), calcium stearate (a lubricant), calcium sulfate, acacia, white wax, carnauba wax, sesame oil (polishing), Blue Dye No. 2, Yellow Dye No. 5, Yellow Dye No. 6, titanium dioxide, polyvinyl pyrolidine, and edible white ink.[2]

Many of these substances cause allergic reactions in susceptible individuals even in such minute amounts. So-called natural vitamins also contain many excipients and additives. While some of these are made from vegetable sources, one can develop susceptibilities to them as well. In general, I urge patients to get their needed vitamins through eating wholesome foods in rotation, according to the principles of the Rotary Diversified Diet (Chap. 18).

The first examination of the role of additives in drug reactions was carried out by Dr. Stephen D. Lockey of the Lancaster General Hospital in 1948. Dr. Lockey reported four cases of hives and three cases of asthma caused by additives in drugs. Lockey's patients became sick when they were given various pharmaceutical preparations which contained petrochemical products. When they were given pure preparations, without these petrochemical additives, they did not become sick. A 58-year-old woman, for example, with a long history of allergies, had frequent attacks of rash and itching. It was eventually learned that these attacks came within half an hour after she had taken synthetic vitamins and an estrogen, a drug used to counteract the effects of the menopause. The only thing that the two capsules had in common was that they both contained Yellow Dye No. 5, a Food and Drug Administration approved coloring. When this patient washed the dye off the two capsules, she was able to use the pills without trouble.

Another patient, a 53-year-old man, took one teaspoonful of elixir of phenobarbital. This brought on an attack of itching, hives, and swelling around the mouth. The drug preparation was colored with the now-banned Red Dye No. 2. In fact, any drug or food containing this dye brought on the same symptoms. The man was able, however, to take sodium phenobarbital tablets without trouble, since the pill form of the drug did not contain any dye.[3]

These are not isolated cases. In my first study of this topic in 1952, I found that over fifty percent of chemically susceptible patients reacted to aspirin and that, in a slightly different group, fifty percent reacted to sulfonamide. This was before the extent of the chemical-susceptibility problem had been worked out and, in particular, before the natural-gas problem was realized to exist. Most chemically susceptible patients are susceptible to synthetic drugs and, in general, the more advanced and long-standing the problem, the greater the number of drugs which are related to such problems.

Although it is best to obtain vitamins from fresh organic food, it should be noted that chemically susceptible patients who take supplements generally react worse to synthetically derived vitamins than to those of natural origin. This is so despite the fact that the two substances seem to have identical chemical structures. Vitamins prepared from food sources may also cause allergic reactions. For instance, Vitamin B_1 prepared from wheat often reacts specifically. Vitamin C may cause reactions in some patients allergic to corn, as the synthetic product is made from corn sugar.

In sum, reactions to drugs in susceptible people may occur to the active chemical ingredients, their bases, artificial colors, scents, preservatives, or other chemical ingredients or contaminants. In view of the number of such possibilities, involving both synthetic and natural ingredients, it is often difficult to trace reactions to the responsible material or materials. At times, combinations of ingredients and circumstances give rise to reactions.

Biological Drugs

Biological drugs are pharmaceuticals made from natural materials. These would seem, at first glance, to be safe for chemically susceptible patients. Yet in some cases they are as bad as synthetic substances.

Susceptibility to biological drugs is a problem which allergists see fairly often but frequently do not know how to interpret. The patient gradually develops strange symptoms, months or even years after beginning a course of antiallergy injections with biologically derived drugs. These reactions continue or get worse following each injection, even when the doctor reduces the potency of the dose. Quite commonly the physician concludes that the patient is a hypochondriac, complaining about the alleged side effects for psychological reasons. The problem is usually chemical, however.

In the early 1950s, several patients became ill each time I tried to give them provocative skin tests with food extracts (see Chap. 16). One patient had no skin reaction to this test but suffered rapidly progressing headaches, nausea, dizziness, and faintness immediately after four injections.

Suspecting some sort of chemical susceptibility, I found that the food extracts which I was using in the tests were preserved with phenol, a coal-tar derived chemical, otherwise known as carbolic acid. (This is the same common chemical also found in the lining of food cans.) Some food extracts without phenol were therefore prepared. The same patients had no adverse reactions to these samples. This test was performed blind, as well; in other words, patients were alternately given phenol-containing and phenol-free injections of the same substance, without knowing which was which. Invariably they became ill from the phenol-containing solution, but not from the phenol-free one. Dr. Jerome Glaser of Rochester, New York, made similar observations, independently, at about the same time.[4]

For many years I maintained a set of phenol-free food extracts for the diagnosis of patients susceptible to this form of the chemical problem. In recent years, far-advanced and complicated cases have been better handled in a hospital setting (Chap. 17).

Reactions to other biological drugs, such as insulin, liver extract, epinephrine, and so forth, can also be traced in many cases to the preservatives in the drug. This can be troublesome indeed, for drugs such as epinephrine, a hormone of the adrenal gland, will rapidly disintegrate without a preservative.

Cosmetics and Perfumes

Closely related to the drug problem is that posed by cosmetics. In fact, as far as the majority of chemically susceptible persons are concerned, the scent of cosmetics is one of the most troublesome features of this problem.

One patient found that she had difficulty riding in elevators or dining out in many restaurants because of her great susceptibility to scents. Sometimes it is only particular perfumes which the susceptible person finds annoying or even suffocating. The safest thing, however, is for such individuals to avoid all perfumes, either on themselves or when worn by others. (The same advice applies to after-shave lotions and colognes, which can be equally irritating to certain individuals.)

Another possible solution is to use only cosmetics and ointments made up entirely of natural ingredients, without artificial colors, scents, and preservatives. Such preparations are more widely available now than they were a decade ago, although use of the word *hypoallergenic* is no guarantee that the product will not cause adverse reactions. Some genuinely nonallergenic products must be refrigerated, since they contain no artificial preservatives.

Reactions to cosmetics, it should be emphasized, usually occur in the presence of an overall susceptibility to the chemical environment. The inability to tolerate these agents alone is rare. More typical is the case of Nora Barnes, discussed in Chapter 3, whose generalized chemical problem was aggravated by her job as a cosmetics salesperson and her own copious use of these products.

The overall question of drug and cosmetic sensitivity is one which has received far too little publicity in recent years. In fact, it has required a struggle even to get the facts about *acute* drug side effects to the public. Yet the question of *chronic*, disguised, long-term harm may be more important than the more dramatic short-term problems caused by these agents.

Since the drug side of this problem is largely caused by the medical profession, supported by the pharmaceutical manufacturers, it is a highly controversial question. And since it involves multiple symptoms, based on an individual's unique reactions to his overall chemical (and food) intake, it is not given to mass-applicable solutions. The existence of this drug susceptibility problem highlights the pressing need for a thoroughly new orientation in medical care, employing more individualized approaches to chronic illness.

6
Indoor Air Pollution

It may have occurred to the reader that air pollution plays a role in the problem of chemical susceptibility. This is true, but not in the way most people suspect. For while it is true that outdoor, or ambient, air pollution is a significant source of exposure, a far greater threat is posed by the presence of indoor, or domiciliary, air pollution.

Indoor air pollution? The term itself is unfamiliar and strange to most people, who tend to think of air pollution solely in terms of smog. Yet the home itself generates combustion products or is directly exposed to them, and many household products give off noxious fumes.

Indoor air pollution is particularly dangerous because exposure to it is so constant. Outdoor air pollution comes and goes; indoor pollution is ever-present, and thus its effects generally remain well hidden. In this it obviously resembles food allergy: as has been explained, allergy to uncommonly eaten foods is readily detected; the real danger comes from allergy to the ordinary foods which we take for granted.

My involvement with the problem of indoor air pollution dates from my earliest chemical-susceptibility cases. In the case of Nora Barnes, for instance, pine paneling and other pine products were implicated as a source of chronic illness. In Ellen Sanders' case, natural gas and pesticide spray resulted in asthma, arthritis, and a host of other complaints. Removal of these pollutants has resulted in her enjoying reasonably good health over a twenty-five-year period.

I first discussed the topic of indoor air pollution in a series of articles published in 1961 and then in my book, *Human Ecology and Susceptibility to the Chemical Environment* (1962). Shortly afterward, the topic became a matter of public debate. In 1962, the government called a conference on air pollution, the first of its kind, in Washington, D.C. As often happens with such conferences, the program and speakers' list were announced first, and then the public was invited to attend. Out of a three-day program, only one-and-a-half hours were allocated for open discussion. During the discussion, I rose to say how astounded I was that no reference had been made, in three days of speeches, to indoor air pollution as a separate topic. In my clinical experience, I added, indoor air pollution was *eight to ten times* more important as a source of chronic illness in susceptible people than ambient air pollution. Outdoor air pollution, I told the gathering, tended to be intermittent and variable, while indoor air pollution was constant. This very constancy made it a source of chronic disease. And of the various materials found in the home, the gas kitchen range, I said, was easily the worst offender.

This left some of the experts without words, but on the far side of the room a gentleman rose and confirmed what I had said, adding some telling details of his own. He introduced himself as Francis Silver. He was an engineer from West Virginia, and later became a member of the Society for Clinical Ecology. We had never met before, but he and I had come to almost identical conclusions about the danger of indoor air pollution, as the result of very different experience—he as an engineer of buildings and I as a clinician studying the effects of such buildings on individual health.

In the following years, there were two conferences devoted solely to the topic of indoor air pollution. In general, these were productive, and I spoke at both.

Since the early 1950s, the extent of the problem of indoor air pollution has continued to grow larger. At the present time, it represents a major source of chronic illness among susceptible individuals in the United States. This can be best understood by considering the kinds of exposures which most frequently result in such chronic health problems.

Fuels, and Their Combustion Products

FUELS

In recent years, energy policy has become a prominent topic of debate. What is almost never taken into account is the long-term harmful effects of petrochemical fuels on susceptible individuals.

The odors of various hydrocarbon fuels such as coal, gasoline, and natural gas can be a source of chronic illness for certain people. Prolonged exposure to such odors or even to their undetected fumes can result in a full spectrum of diseases.

Some of the worst practices of the past are now gone. In the old days, for instance, when coal was delivered by chute to the basement of one's house, kerosene was often sprayed on the coal to control dust. It slowly gave off fumes, contaminating the basement or dwelling.

Today, fuel oil and natural gas have replaced coal and wood in most areas. These can give rise to their own set of problems, however. Old oil tanks, for instance, may leak and give off fumes which are almost imperceptible to those who have lived in the house for a while. With oil, there is always the danger of an overflow while the tanks are being filled. If a basement floor has been flooded with fuel oil, the odor tends to remain for several months or even years, despite the best cleanup efforts. This has caused numerous problems for susceptible individuals; in a few cases they have been forced to abandon their homes entirely.

Most fuel-oil installations, whether furnaces or space heaters, give off a characteristic odor. Although they tend to smell worse when they are actually operating, there may be enough odor coming from them even when they are shut down to cause reactions in highly susceptible patients.

Natural gas is advertised as the "clean fuel." This may be so from the point of view of visible or smog-producing residues, but for the chemically susceptible individual this gas may be the worst form of fuel.

In the early part of this century, most cities were supplied with artificial gas derived from coal. Especially after World War Two, with the completion of a national gas line network, most cities switched to natural gas. From the point of view of chronic disease, it does not really matter whether artificial or natural gas is used, since both can cause problems for those with the chemical problem. Natural gas, however, is delivered at much higher pressures than the artificial product. This, in turn, can cause a serious problem of leakage if the pipes were originally constructed for the transmission of artificial gas. In Chicago, for instance, joints and turns in the old gas line become potential or actual sources of leakage. Gas, being lighter than air, tends to rise from the basement or kitchen into the rest of the house. The greater the amount of piping and the number of outlets, and the more pilots and other automatic devices on gas appliances, the greater will be the probability of leaks.

Perhaps one of the most surprising aspects of this gas problem is the incredible sensitivity of some people to its presence. Merely shutting off a gas range is not enough to bring relief to such patients. The gas stove must be *completely removed* from the premises. This is because even a non-working range continues to give off odors from the gas which it has absorbed over the years.

In the course of my practice, I have directed almost 3,000 patients to remove their gas kitchen ranges because I found these people to be susceptible to chemical odors and fumes. This decision was not taken lightly or on the basis of blind hunch but after scientific tests, such as those conducted in the Ecology Unit (Chap. 17). To date, none of these patients has complained that the changeover was not worth the cost or trouble.

In many cases, in fact, when the range was removed for the benefit of one member of the family, other members of the family also reported an improvement in health. A gas range was removed from the home of one patient, a girl with persistent headaches. Her mother, who was not a patient, reported an unsuspected benefit, however. While cooking with gas, she had often become highly irritable. She would scream at the children or anyone else who came into "her kitchen." Since she frequently had a kitchen knife in her hand when she started screaming, this frightened the children and created a bad atmosphere at dinnertime. With the removal of the gas range, her temper tantrums quickly subsided. What had appeared to be a potential "mental" problem was solved simply by removing a hidden environmental pollutant.

In cases in which actual removal of the gas range has been impossible, certain halfway measures have proven useful. They have included increased ventilation of the kitchen; installation of a kitchen door, which is kept closed during the time the stove is on, keeping fumes from reaching the rest of the house; or disconnection of the stove, without actual removal. For many people, such measures are beneficial; for the seriously ill, however, there is no substitute for complete removal of the offending appliance.

COMBUSTION PRODUCTS OF FUELS

Another serious problem is posed by the combustion products of home fuel systems. This source of danger is largely dependent on the type and location of the furnace, rather than on the type of fuel used.

The warm-air furnace is most frequently implicated as the source of chronic illness. When a chemically susceptible patient moves out of a home with such a furnace and into an ecologically sound environment, he often experiences an improvement in health. Returning to the home heated with warm air similarly may result in a decreased level of health.

The furnace of a warm-air system may pollute the air of the basement in which the furnace is located by releasing combustion products each time it is turned on. Leaks in such systems are common, and warm-air furnaces produce more dust and general agitation of the environment than some other types of systems. This is complicated by the fact that the warm-air system *forces* heated air throughout the whole house, thus naturally spreading dust and fumes.

Chemically susceptible people in homes with warm-air heat react with remarkable rapidity to the turning on of the heat. In fact, they begin to develop symptoms more quickly, sometimes, than the fumes could possibly spread from the basement. A psychological reaction? Not necessarily. Upon investigation, it was found that these patients were also susceptible to dust, a common source of allergic reactions; any dust which landed on the hot furnace was burned and then spewed in minute particles around the house. This "fried dust" was then stirred up every time the furnace was activated, and spread more quickly than the fumes.

The location of the furnace can be particularly important. A person who lives directly above a furnace is more likely to feel its effects than one who is sleeping in an area removed from the source of heat. The worst housing arrangement is probably the ranch-style house, with the furnace right in the center of the main floor. The next worse is to have an open utility room on the same floor as the living quarters. Either of these designs will subject the inhabitants to a daily dose of pollutants every time the furnace starts up.

Essentially, the only completely safe way to handle a furnace is to put it *outside the house.* It can be placed in a garage, in a separate room between the house and the garage, or in a separate area adjacent to the house which can only be entered from the outside. The only opening between this room and the house itself should be a well-insulated hole through which the hot water or steam pipes pass. Once the heating is thus arranged, it does not really matter if one uses coal, oil, or gas, as long as warm water or steam central heating is employed to convey the heat.

The gas range is the most common source of indoor pollution, but the most dangerous is probably the unvented gas-burning room wall-heater. Although this pernicious device is becoming less common, it is still found throughout the American Southwest. It is certainly ironic that people like Ellen Sanders should flee to the land of sunshine only to find a worse source of pollution in their new homes.[1]

Paint, Varnish, and Solvents

Another major source of indoor air pollution is the odor or fumes of paint, varnish, and other solvents. Conventional allergists have long known that the odors of these substances could bring on attacks of bronchial asthma. The effects of such agents on chemically susceptible persons go far beyond this, however, and cover the gamut of physical and so-called mental diseases.

If a person is highly aware of the odor of paint, this is a blessing, since he may know enough to avoid such odors and their effects. Some patients are so acutely aware of it that they can enter a high-rise apartment or office building, take one whiff, and announce that painting is going on. In actuality, the painting may be taking place many stories above them, but they can detect even the faintest traces of odor.

For many people, fresh paint constitutes a fairly infrequent exposure; hence it is less of a danger than natural gas, which is ever-present in many households. Sometimes reactions to paint can result in bizarre "mental" symptoms.

Denise Miller was the manager of a large retail store. She worked in the business office of that store, in the rear of the building, adjacent to the parking lot. When she sat near an open window and worked, she inevitably became depressed. The source of her problem was located in the cars and busses which spewed their exhausts in the direction of her office all day long. Since she could not change her place of employment, she was able to get a good deal of relief simply by keeping the windows shut and sitting some distance away from them.

One winter she took her vacation in Florida. Staying with relatives, she was given a big room, with the bed away from the walls of the room. She had no problem. But during the last two days of her stay, other relatives came to visit, and so she was moved into a smaller room with the bed wedged in one corner. The walls of this room, as well as the rest of the house, had been painted not long before, and Miss Miller began to react.

She hallucinated, seeing purple frogs hopping around her room. A lion sat on the foot of her bed and scared her out of her wits. In desperation, she decided to go home. On the Twentieth Century Limited to New York, she later said, she shared her bed with a gorilla. She was very upset, since every time she tried to get to sleep, the gorilla's arms enfolded her!

Tests revealed that these strange symptoms were brought on by exposure to fresh paint, which was part of her overall susceptibility to many chemicals. By avoiding such exposure, she was able to maintain relatively good health.

Cleaning Fluids and Lighter Fluids

Dry cleaning can be a source of trouble for chemically susceptible persons. Clothes which have been dry-cleaned may retain traces of the fluids used by the cleaning establishment. Some dry cleaners now add soil retardants or moth repellants to the dry cleaning fluids. This is a hazardous practice. Some individuals are so susceptible to these agents that they cannot enter or even inhale the air outside of a dry cleaning shop without feeling sick.

Rug cleaners can also be a source of danger, and for this reason rug cleaning must proceed only when a susceptible person is away from home. The fumes should be allowed to evaporate and air out before he returns. Home cleaning agents, including rug cleaners, should be stored outside the house, a point to which we shall return (Chap. 20).

It should be noted that there is an additional unsuspected hazard in over-zealous cleaning of rugs. If the rug or carpet does not dry thoroughly between washings, it makes an ideal environment for molds to grow in. This is especially a danger in hot and humid climates, such as the American South. Molds, as allergy-causing substances, can produce many of the same symptoms as those which are produced by food or chemicals.[2]

Cigarette lighter fluid is similarly dangerous for the susceptible person and should be eliminated from the home.

Refrigerants and Spray Containers

Electric refrigerators cool by means of circulating certain rare refrigerant gases. Air conditioners work on a similar principle. In the course of operation, either through some defect or through wear and tear, the gases can slowly begin to leak out of these appliances. Such leakage can be a major problem for some people, a source of long-term health problems.

Even if you cannot smell these gases, there are ways to detect their presence. If the refrigerator runs constantly, for instance, this may indicate the loss of refrigerant gas. So, too, does a gradually decreasing frosted surface. If a person reacts to food stored or frozen in the refrigerator and does not react to the same lot of food prior to freezing, this is a sign that refrigerator gas may be the health culprit.

The same compressed gas is commonly used as a propellant in spray cans containing insecticides, perfumes, hair sprays, and other cosmetics. Many of these substances can cause health reactions themselves, and so, when he uses these spray cans, the susceptible person is hit by a kind of "double-barreled" barrage. Certain types of foods are also dispensed in pressurized cannisters, especially toppings.

Pesticides

Prominent among the sources of indoor air pollution are the pesticides. These are toxic agents which people introduce into their homes, offices, and neighborhoods for the control of insects or rodents. Since World War Two, there has been an explosive increase in the use of these agents. The foundations of houses are now routinely treated with a powerful insecticide to deter termites. Many persons contract with exterminators for the periodic treatment of their homes. Apartment-dwellers are encouraged, or pressured, by landlords to permit extermination to be done on a periodic basis. External mosquito-abatement programs are carried out in many communities, and rural areas are saturated with farm and forest pesticide programs. To a greater degree than almost anyone realizes, a kind of pesticide fog now hangs over the United States and some of the other industrialized countries.

Yet many people are highly susceptible to these agents. Pesticides are among the leading health dangers for those with the chemical problem. In some cases, exposure to pesticides may trigger acute episodes of distress. Ellen Sanders almost died from a particularly heavy exposure (Chap. 3). Other patients trace the onset of their worst symptoms to massive contact with pesticide spray.

More commonly, undetected, long-term health problems are brought on by daily exposure to spray. Unexplained chronic illnesses develop as a reaction to spray, possibly in combination with other chemical or food susceptibility. A woman with arthritis, for example, will rarely associate her joint pain with the brightly colored fly-killing pest strip hanging in her kitchen. Much less will anyone connect a general feeling of malaise and fatigue with the exterminator who comes knocking once a month.

Once pesticides are applied in the home, it is extremely difficult to remove them. Even minute amounts of residues can perpetuate symptoms. When my special facility, the Ecology Unit, was first set up, in the ward of a hospital, for the diagnosis and treatment of environmental disease, it was found that we could not clear some patients of their symptoms. The difficulty was ultimately traced to the fact that this ward, along with the rest of the hospital, had previously been sprayed with pesticides. The only solution was to rip up the floors and baseboards and replace them with unsprayed materials (Chap. 17). In some extreme instances, patients have had to sell their homes and move, after their dwellings had been carelessly treated with pesticides.

Sponge Rubber

Sponge rubber is another "modern miracle" with unexpected drawbacks. Sponge-rubber pillows, mattresses, upholstery, seat cushions, rug backings, typewriter pads, and certain noise-reducing devices have all been identified as the sources of chronic illness.

Some allergy patients, having substituted sponge rubber for other bedding in order to reduce exposure to household dust, find to their dismay that the rubber fumes are even more troublesome. More commonly the effects of the rubber go undetected.

Frequently, a susceptible person will experience flushing of the face, irritability, and "air hunger," upon first entering a room with rubber rug-pads, upholstery, or rubber-tiled floors. At night, he may suffer from insomnia, restlessness, night sweats, or fatigue, in reaction to rubber pillows, mattresses, or the rubber insulation of electric blankets. Natural fiber substitutes for all of these things are available, however, and their use is essentially the solution to this aspect of the chemical-susceptibility problem.[3]

Plastics

The modern era has sometimes been called the Age of Plastic. Indeed, it is difficult to avoid this almost ubiquitous synthetic material. The threat of indoor air pollution from plastics comes mainly from the "plasticizers" added to make such substances soft, flexible, or resilient. As a general rule, the more easily you can bend a plastic, the more potentially dangerous it is to your health. Another way to sense danger is with your nose: the more odorous the plastic, the more these plasticizers are slipping into the environment.

Hard plastics, such as the older Bakelite and Formica, are, accordingly, rarely incriminated as the cause of chronic illness. The worst offenders are soft materials, such as the plastic used in pillow and mattress cases, upholstery materials, shoes and handbags, and so forth. Naugahyde has been particularly troublesome for some patients. Plastic brushes, combs, powder cases, shoes, and other articles of clothing also occasionally become the source of chronic health problems in patients.

Flexible plastics used in the storage of refrigerated food are particularly menacing. One young child was brought to me for skin problems. It turned out that his mother was a salesperson for a well-known brand of plastic containers. She was shocked when I blamed this product for contributing to her son's skin problems. Elimination of the plastic containers, however, brought a dramatic improvement in his rash, and this woman soon sought another line of work.

Mechanical Devices

Most mechanical devices require petroleum-derived oil as a lubricant. As these machines operate, some of the oil escapes into the air. This atmospheric pollutant may pose a problem for certain people. The most common source of such oil in the home is the air conditioner. The air-conditioning unit not only emits a "normal" amount of oil as it runs but generally has an oil-impregnated glass-wool or fiber filter. Some patients who were affected by air conditioners have been able to use the appliance with impunity when unoiled filters were substituted.

Kitchen devices with motors may be another source of indoor air pollution. These time-saving appliances are proliferating, often without a thought being given to their possible drawbacks. If a refrigerator, food processor, electric hand beater, can opener, and air conditioner are all operating in a kitchen, this can represent a considerable source of oil fumes. In addition, it should be noted that such electric motors emit minute amounts of ozone, a rare form of oxygen, which is highly toxic. American and Soviet scientists have found that humans may be endangered by exposure to fifty parts per billion of ozone in the atmosphere. Susceptible persons may be even more likely to incur damage from ozone in a closed environment.[4]

Automobiles

It may seem surprising to include the automobile as a source of indoor air pollution. Yet, not only does ambient (outdoor) air pollution enter the home, but the automobile itself has become part of the home in parts of the United States. Many houses have been built with the garage incorporated into their structures. This is particularly true in the case of ranch houses. Not uncommonly, the master bedroom is located directly above the garage and is saturated by fumes rising from it.

For the chemically susceptible, this development in modern living can be disastrous. Simply stated, garages should not be incorporated into the basements of homes unless elaborate precautions are taken to prevent fumes and odors from rising and fouling the air of the living quarters. To do this, however, is extremely difficult—in fact, nearly impossible. Even a passageway between a garage and home may allow sufficient fumes to enter the house to cause or perpetuate symptoms. Careless home construction often contributes to this problem.

A similar situation prevails in many apartment houses, where garage fumes get into the elevator shafts and contaminate the living quarters of the buildings. One partial solution to this problem is to let a car cool off completely before putting it into the garage. In this way, engine fumes will be less apt to accumulate and pollute the house.

CASE STUDY: CHEMICAL SUSCEPTIBILITY

Sister Francesca came to me with a peculiar complaint. She suffered from aches and pains in her rib cage, on both sides, about six inches below her armpits. While aches and pains are commonly the result of allergylike problems, there were no organs in that particular part of the body which would be likely to give rise to them. I was confused, more so when I noticed that her associate, who had accompanied her to the doctor, was fighting back a smile as the sister related her problem.

I later found out the reason for the strange soreness: the sister had a habit of falling asleep every morning at Mass. As she began to snore, her fellow nuns on either side would crack her in the ribs with their elbows to wake her up again. This went on repeatedly during Mass, giving rise to her medical complaint.

Upon inquiry, I found that the chapel of her convent was directly over the garage which held the community's five automobiles. I therefore arranged with the priests who drove these cars to leave all of them outside for a week and leave the doors of the garage wide open. They were sworn to secrecy, however, and Sister Francesca was never told anything about this arrangement.

That week, Sister Francesca attended Mass as usual, but was alert and awake all week, with no snoring and no sore ribs. Then, again without telling her, the priests were instructed to resume parking the cars in the garage with the door closed. On the next morning, Sister Francesca entered the chapel, took her seat, and promptly fell asleep. The other nuns awakened her as she began to snore.

It was a very convincing experiment, and from that point on the automobiles were kept outside the incriminated garage.

Miscellaneous Indoor Pollutants

Inhalation of the odors and fumes of detergents, soaps containing naptha, ammonia, Clorox, cleansing powders containing bleaches, window-washing compounds, certain silver- and brass-polishing materials, and burning wax candles may all cause chronic or acute symptoms. Even merely storing bleach-containing cleansers in the house has caused problems for some people.

Soap can be very irritating, although in general susceptible individuals have shown much greater tolerance for unscented soaps and cleansers than for highly scented soaps, toilet deodorants, and disinfectants, especially pine-scented ones. So-called air fresheners and improvers, which evaporate in the air, are particularly troublesome. Other patients have reported reacting to the odor of highly scented perfumes or other cosmetics.

Even the odor arising from prolonged use of television sets has been enough to foul the air in the vicinity, since the plastic-coated hot wires give off fumes.

In short, chemicals and plastics have been introduced into the home to a prodigious degree in the last few decades. Products made from these materials have often represented a boon, in that they are cheap, readily manufactured in large quantities, and capable of functions which could not be so well performed by the natural products which they have replaced. They have also made a great deal of money for their manufacturers and suppliers.

What has almost never been considered has been the long-range health consequences of these new materials. It was simply assumed that these bountiful results of scientific progress were as good for us as they were convenient. This conviction has turned out to be profoundly wrong. Many of the substances naively welcomed into the home have turned into hidden enemies, polluting our environment and the very air we breathe.

In recent years, for example, formaldehyde has been increasingly implicated as a source of allergy-type reactions. In March of 1980 the prestigious National Academy of Sciences concluded that formaldehyde, even at low levels, did indeed pose a serious health problem.

Formaldehyde is found in such diverse products as home-heating insulation, plywood, particleboard, permanent-press clothes, toothpaste, air fresheners, shampoo, and cosmetics, as previously mentioned.

According to the Academy report, formaldehyde, "even at extremely low airborne concentrations," will irritate the eyes, nose, and throat of a proportion of the public. One-fifth of the entire population, in fact, is affected to some degree by the presence of this chemical.[5]

In my experience, the Academy may be understating the seriousness of this growing problem. I, and other clinical ecologists, have seen patients literally forced from their homes by formaldehyde exposure.

Public Places

The same problems encountered in the home are also found in public places, sometimes to a greater degree. Deodorants, disinfectants, pine-scented sweeping compounds, and insect sprays are commonly encountered. How distressing it is, for instance, to enter a public toilet only to find it thoroughly polluted with some pine- or artificial "fruit"-scented deodorant. Acute reactions of patients after such encounters are becoming increasingly common.

Fuel-oil or gas space-heaters are also found more often in small shops, stores, and restaurants than in homes; these can be major causes of *chronic* reactions in workers and of *acute* responses in customers. One patient, for instance, tells of going to dinner at a small Italian restaurant. She had to change her seat a number of times because of currents of gas coming from a space heater in the kitchen every time the kitchen door swung open. Even so, she suffered familiar symptoms that evening, a kind of "spaciness" in her brain, followed by headache, which she often experienced after encountering natural gas.

Schools

One of the most disturbing aspects of the indoor air pollution problem is the involvement of schools. Here, the use of various chemicals can contribute to the overall chemical and food problem to cause poor performance by both children and teachers.

Poorly designed heating and cooking systems in schools are a major source of trouble. One teacher was always dopey and drowsy when he taught a class located directly above the school cafeteria, from which gas-range odors emanated. His performance improved dramatically when he transferred to a more distant room.

Children suffer all sorts of adverse reactions to chemicals in school, including hyperactivity, inattention, irritability, and the like. This is especially so among children addicted to "junk food," who live in a polluted home environment.

In 1967, Mrs. Kathleen A. Blume carried out with my help a study of indoor air pollution at a public school in Wauconda, Illinois, a suburb of Chicago.[6] Mrs. Blume, a home economics teacher, was aided by local parents who were concerned about the quality of air in their children's schools.

They literally sniffed out problems in the schools:

> We used both eyes and nose searching and sniffing our way through . . . school trying to uncover the elusive as well as glaring causes of air contamination. In spite of advances in instruments for measuring contaminating particulates in the air, the human nose remains the chief detector of offensive odors.

It is remarkable, and depressing, how many sources of air pollution these parents were able to find stored in the school. For example, aerosol sprays are known to cause problems because of their volatile mixtures of chemicals, solvents, and the propellant, Freon (itself a mixture of carbon, chlorine, and flourine). The parents found insecticide sprays; paint, enamel, and lacquer sprays; fixatives; spray snow; spray plastic; solvent cleaner; germicidal cleaners; room deodorants; hair spray; furniture polish; disinfectants; deodorants; and even fungicidal sprays for the locker room.

Francis Silver, the engineer who studied this list and cooperated in the Wauconda study, reported that none of these, with the possible exception of the spray enamel and the fixative, could be justified from an ecological point of view.

In some cases, the children were more aware of the dangers of the sprays than the adults. One child, for instance, complained of a burning sensation in her nose, eyes, and throat after a janitor sprayed a disinfectant in a room full of children. This child's problem lasted well into the evening. When a teacher cleaned her desk top with a spray cleaner, one of the children disliked the smell so much that he asked permission to leave the room. And when another teacher sprayed fixative on chalk drawings, several children complained of the odor and asked her to open the windows.

It should be noted that such sprays not only pose a danger of provoking allergylike symptoms but can result in "spray keratitis," or damage to the sensitive cornea of the eye from chemical particles in aerosol spray cans.[7]

Another source of problems in the Wauconda study was janitorial supplies. Twenty-eight different chemicals were found in the supply closets, including some highly toxic products. Mrs. Blume commented:

> Janitorial supplies are probably the saddest part of the story. Janitorial chemicals receive no supervision, anything goes. We are so particular about who is allowed to prescribe drugs for patients but janitors spread their products around which then evaporate into the breathed air and are then ingested. . . . If we were more interested in health and not just in treatment, we would probably be more particular about our janitors than we are about our physicians.

The use of such products in schools often represents an "overkill" of bacteria. Dr. Malcolm Hargraves, a senior consultant at the Mayo Clinic, has said:

> The American people, I am afraid, are greatly oversold by any article which makes the claim that it is medicated [i.e., anti-bacterial]. The universal use of such agents with such an idea only leads to the development of more resistant strains of bacteria to plague us in the future.[8]

Actually, fresh air, sunshine, hot water, and unscented soap are still the best disinfecting agents. The "progress" in inventing disinfectants of the last thirty or forty years has added little to our ability to control infectious diseases, while piling up problems for the chemically susceptible. It is tragic to expose children to these and other agents so early, creating a problem which may remain with them for the rest of their lives.

Other Public Places

Few studies of public places have been as complete as this parents' report from Wauconda. Similar findings would undoubtedly be made, however, at other schools, universities, laboratories, offices, and hospitals.

Each public place has its own potential dangers. Offices, for example, often contain a variety of possible irritants, including carbon paper, ink, mimeographing and duplicating devices, rubber cement, typewriters, typewriter pads, plastic lamps and fixtures, and perfumes and scents. The new type of carbonless carbon paper is particularly troublesome to many patients. If the office is new, the odor of freshly chemicalized carpet is often strong. Some offices are adjacent to factories, warehouses, shops, and garages, and share a common heating and ventilation system with them. Many people who are susceptible to chemicals are also affected by tobacco smoke, which can reach heavy concentration in some offices.

Hospitals, on the other hand, have their own peculiar smells: deodorants, disinfectants, and cleansers; ether fumes and other anesthetics from the operating room; odors of drugs and rubbing alcohol; and the smell of rubber draw-sheets and plastic bedding material.

As I have pointed out, the air of supermarkets is often fouled by the odors of insecticides, disinfectants, deodorants, and the like. A peculiar odor often emanates from the freezer sections, sometimes as the result of leaking refrigerants. Ammonia is frequently used in cleaning refrigerators, often while customers are still in the store.

Even churches provide no sanctuary for the chemically susceptible. Gas is often detectable, coming from a well-hidden kitchen. There is also the odor of burning candles (in recent years, mainly petroleum-based rather than made of bees' wax), incense, perfumes, and the mothball-like smell of furs and outer garments.

Finally, a word should be said about pollution inside factories, although this enormous topic falls outside the scope of this book. In factories, many of the already-mentioned pollutants are mixed with the special odors which arise from manufacturing and processing. The worst offenders tend to be solvents and their combustion products: rubber, plastic, resins, detergents, cutting and lubricating oils, sulfur, chlorine, and similar agents. Large-scale outbreaks of illness have already taken place in electronic plants and other plants where such materials are handled. While traditionalists have ascribed this to "mass psychogenic illness," some environmental health experts have interpreted it as a sign of chemical susceptibility on the part of large numbers of workers.[9]

7

Outdoor Air Pollution

Although indoor air pollution is the more serious source of reactions for the chemically susceptible, one should not minimize the danger of outdoor, or ambient, sources of pollution.

Outdoor air pollution is by its very nature variable and intermittent. That is, the intensity of the "smog" frequently depends on local weather conditions. In general, the worst spells of outdoor air pollution occur during stagnant, humid, foggy, or rainy days. This type of weather is apt to be more common in winter. Summer has its own problems, too, with more cars on the road giving off copious fumes from their overheated engines.

Chicago is a particularly good city in which to study this problem. As a storm approaches from the west, air pollution is swept into the city, from the industrial center in the south, by the counterclockwise winds swirling around a low pressure area. When the storm center passes through the city, the winds shift suddenly to the north and east, which clears the air of its major pollutants. Thus, both pollution and the lack of pollution are sharply accentuated by the geography of this area.

Chicago contains four major sources of outdoor air pollution. The greatest is the petroleum refinery area at the extreme northern border of Illinois and Indiana. The reader will recall Nora Barnes' onset of sickness upon driving through the smog of this industrial zone. Some patients from Michigan prefer to take the ferry from Ludington to Milwaukee and then drive down to Chicago from the north, simply to avoid passing through the area.

The second major source of pollution comes from a refinery area adjoining the ship canal, southwest of Chicago. A third, more diffuse source centers around a paint manufacturing plant on the south side, which is located near several other foci of heavy industry.

The fourth area is the Loop, Chicago's famous business district. Here automobile and railroad odors are major pollutants. Expressways and diesel railways radiate, spokelike, from the Loop, spewing chemical contamination into the environment.

Depending on the direction and force of the winds, pollutants from these four sources frequently mingle in a noxious cloud, and the contaminated blanket of air they have created is pushed now in one direction, now another. Hardly anyone can escape the influence of this smog, although the south side of the city usually suffers the most, and the lakeside "Gold Coast" the least.

CASE STUDY: CHEMICAL SUSCEPTIBILITY

Patrick Wells, an architect, had a long history of medical problems, including running nose (rhinitis), coughing, headache, fatigue, mental confusion, and intermittent bouts of depression. Like many people in Chicago, he worked in the Loop and commuted by rail to a suburb west of the city. Under my care, he had already controlled various aspects of indoor air pollution in his home, yet many of his symptoms persisted. Suspecting that there was a relationship between the weather and his problems, he kept a log of all of his symptoms for each day, and of the weather conditions prevailing on that day. He carefully monitored this for a year, without missing a day. He also obtained data from the United States Weather Bureau concerning wind velocity and visibility on these days.

Wells found that he was, in effect, a "human barometer." At both home and work, he remained symptom-free on those days when the wind blew from the west, northwest, and north (there is little industry in these regions). Invariably, however, his depression and other symptoms returned when the wind blew from the east, and particularly from the southeast. This, of course, is where the heavy industry is located, especially the refineries and largest industrial plants. Winds from the south and even the southwest were also troublesome.

It was particularly interesting that Wells had no trouble from *any* wind with a velocity of fifteen or more miles per hour. The pollution, apparently, had to *drift* slowly over the area at a leisurely three to seven miles per hour in order to affect him.

Wells' observations were later confirmed by other chemically susceptible patients in Chicago. It was always the slow, southern winds that brought with them symptom-causing pollution. In particular, as Wells found, the severity of such effects could be correlated with the visibility factor (visibility being defined as the distance one is able to see spaced lights). The lesser the visibility, the greater the chance of chronic symptoms on any particular day.

Further incidents revealed the remarkable carrying power of these slowly drifting winds, and how they could bring pollution to the doorstep of unsuspecting people many miles away.

One day, in the Chicago area, a number of my chemically susceptible patients became acutely ill at the same time. Several of them claimed to smell refinery odors in the air, although they did not live near refineries. Plotting their homes on a map and studying weather patterns for that day, I concluded that these people were reacting to chemical "fallout" from the Joliet refineries, although they all lived in the northern suburbs of Chicago, forty to seventy-five miles away.

Many similar incidents have occurred over the years. Even the northernmost suburbs of Chicago, near the Wisconsin border, occasionally receive some of the air pollution from Chicago's south side. In fact, there is no residential area within a fifty- to seventy-five-mile radius of the center of Chicago which is consistently free of air pollution from the city or its industrial locales. The same is true of many American cities.

Engine Exhausts

For the chemically susceptible, the worst kind of engine exhaust is that of diesels. Diesel exhaust is particularly aggravating to many susceptible individuals and if encountered in the course of driving can represent a real traffic hazard.

Busses using diesel fuel can be troublesome for passengers or those riding in other vehicles. Moving vehicles generally tend to suck in their own exhaust fumes if the windows are open. Therefore if a passenger rides in the rear of the bus, he is more likely to be exposed to these fumes than if he stays in the front of the passenger compartment. One patient with a relatively mild form of the chemical-susceptibility problem reported that he enjoyed riding in the back of the bus with the window open. He found this a stimulating experience, although he had no idea why. Afterwards, however, he noticed a feeling of depression. This appears to have been an addictionlike response to chemical fumes.

Sometimes busses follow each other in a caravan. In these cases, the exhaust of one bus is swept up into the passenger compartment of the next, especially if the wind is traveling in the same direction as the fumes.

Passengers often develop headaches and other reactions, such as nausea, during or following bus trips, without ever suspecting exhaust fumes as the cause. These effects can be cumulative, occurring after the passengers have been riding in the vehicle for a certain number of miles or minutes. In less susceptible people, the symptoms may only come on if the bus is in poor repair or if the rear windows are left open.

Often the effects of diesel fumes are subtle and go unnoticed. For instance, the fatigue associated with riding the bus downtown to go shopping is frequently out of proportion to the actual amount of activity involved. Much of this exhaustion often stems from the fumes of busses and from general traffic pollution.

In railroad stations, the diesel fumes are greatest at the entrances and exits. This is especially true of underground or covered stations in which passengers are forced to walk past a line of "purring" locomotives to reach their coach or the station exit. Some patients have become acutely ill whenever they have attempted to run such a gauntlet. Other than this, however, diesel trains actually provide less troublesome exposure than busses or automobiles, especially during rush-hour traffic. The reason for this is the rapid speed of the trains, the avoidance of traffic jams, and the relative isolation of the passenger compartment from the source of pollution.

Other Exhausts

"Normal" car exhaust, dispensed by automobiles into the general environment, is a major source of air pollution and of chronic health problems. In Chicago, this foul air is generated by the heavy traffic in the downtown area. From here, following the spokelike course of railroad tracks, truck routes, bus lines, expressways, and other highways, contaminated air radiates out to the open countryside and also criss-crosses the entire metropolitan area. Because vehicles move more slowly there, and decrease their speed more frequently, railway stations and traffic stops tend to be "hot spots" of pollution.

I usually urge patients not to buy a home or rent an apartment near a major intersection or a main thoroughfare. Diesel railroads, truck, or bus lines are also to be avoided. Living three blocks from a major highway has, in some instances, been enough to promote chronic symptoms. As a general rule, if one can hear the roar of traffic, one is too close for comfort.

Car Sickness

It is a common observation that automobile passengers are far less likely to become sick if they ride in the front rather than in the rear of the passenger compartment. In fact, moving to the front seat is the traditional "cure" for car sickness. But why is that?

One reason is that the rear passengers are exposed to more air pollution than those in the front. If the rear windows or station-wagon "gate" are open even a crack, exhaust fumes from the car will enter the rear seating area. This is because a car in motion creates a vacuum behind it, and the vacuum sucks exhausts into the passenger compartment. The location of the exhaust pipe to the side of some cars helps the problem but does not solve it. It should be noted that car sickness is not the same as motion sickness. This is shown by the fact that many people become sick while riding in cars who are not affected by trips in other conveyances, such as electrically propelled busses or trains.

Other forms of car-induced problems include "driver hypnosis." This is the onset of fatigue and overpowering sleepiness which occurs after several hours of driving. Often the physical fatigue of driving and of staring at the road is heightened by the more subtle effect of exhaust fumes. People driving under the influence of fumes may find their ability to make quick decisions diminished and their tolerance for other drivers decreased, which can result in extremely hostile and violent behavior. If the driver is a "food-a-holic," frequent stops at junk-food dispensaries along the highway will not improve his behavior.

In addition, massive exposures to chemicals commonly encountered along the road can result in immediate, acute symptoms. These include fresh road tar, car exhausts, pesticide sprays, and airport pollution. This usually involves some impairment in muscle coordination, nervousness, tenseness, blurring of vision, and so forth. The afflicted driver rarely understands the cause of his "attack of nerves." Sometimes chemical reactions progress to the point of apparent "drunkenness," although the driver has not had anything inebriating to drink.

Alcoholics may be unable to tell the location of their feet unless they first look at them. Drivers in the "drunken" stage of chemical reactivity similarly cannot tell how much force they are applying to either the gas or the brake pedal unless they look. And looking, of course, adds to the danger, since now the driver's eyes are not on the road. Some patients, such as Ida Koller (Chap. 1), have been pulled off the road in such a condition and forced to take a breath test by the police, only to pass it, to the confusion and consternation of the officers. Some drivers may realize that something is going wrong and turn the wheel over to someone else or pull over to the side of the road. Some victims smash up their cars and those of others, never knowing the true cause of their bizarre behavior. One wonders how many of the thousands of "unexplained" automobile accidents are helped along by acute reactions to pollution.

What has been said about drivers also applies to pedestrians. A person on foot, wading through a blanket of smog, may temporarily become thoroughly confused and lose all perception of danger. Stand at a busy intersection sometime during a smog alert and watch the pedestrians. Seemingly normal people often walk like zombies in such situations, impervious to danger. In fact, in smoggy situations a driver cannot assume a normal degree of perception and awareness on the part of any pedestrian. I once saw one of my patients trying to cross a downtown street: he began to cross with the light, got half-way across, stopped, and then crossed back again in a daze. Further investigation showed that he was not simply lost, but was benumbed by the outdoor air pollution.

The automobile has been called the focus of our civilization, and has certainly transformed our lives, making transportation both more convenient and more pleasant, in many cases. But we are also discovering many drawbacks to this mode of transportation, including unsuspected acute and chronic health problems. The added load which the automobile adds to our chemical-susceptibility problem is certainly one of its major deficits.

CASE STUDY: CHEMICAL SUSCEPTIBILITY (AIR POLLUTION)

Theodore Muysenberg came to me with a suspected dust allergy. He was treated with extracts of house dust, a procedure commonly employed to desensitize patients to this source of allergic reaction. Soon after receiving his injection, however, he would be overcome with headache and fatigue and would have to lie down in my office until the reaction wore off.

Since some patients react to the chemical preservative used in the preparation of house-dust extract, Muysenberg was given a chemical-free preparation. Again, however, he became acutely ill. On the next visit the dose was reduced, on the theory that the amount given, although very small, may have been the source of the reaction. Again, he became ill.

Since he lived outside the city, these trips to Chicago were becoming a burden for him, but in an effort to get to the bottom of his reaction, he continued to come. Nothing seemed to work, or rather, *everything* seemed to bring on these distressing symptoms.

As a control test, Muysenberg was given an injection of preservative-free normal saline solution, which generally has no effect on the body at all. Again, however, he suffered his characteristic fatigue and headaches. After a few hours, he was given another appointment and sent home. The next time, he was jabbed in the arm with a *dry* needle. This time, too, he became tired, headachey, and had to lie down. The next time he came, he was given *no* injection at all: he was simply sent home without any treatment and told to watch for symptoms. A few hours later he called and said that he had developed the familiar symptoms on the trip back.

At this point, of course, many doctors would have referred this patient to a psychiatrist or attributed his symptoms to the strain of his intellectually demanding job. Having been alerted by the experience of other patients, however, I thought to ask Muysenberg what means of transportation he used to get to my office and to return home. The bus, he answered. I therefore "prescribed" the elevated train for his next trip into town.

This time there was no headache, exhaustion, or any untoward reaction at all. Muysenberg was able to take his dust-allergy injections with impunity and to return home with no problem, provided that he used the "El." Whenever he attempted to ride the diesel-powered bus for any length of time, however, the same distressing symptoms returned—symptoms which, in other circumstances, might have landed him on a psychiatrist's couch.

Another patient got abdominal cramps and diarrhea whenever she attempted to ride a few blocks on a diesel bus but was able to ride several *miles* on a propane-fueled bus before the same symptoms came on. Sleepiness and mental confusion are reactions which are also often seen among chemically susceptible bus riders.

Fogging for Insect Abatement and Weed Control

We have spoken of insecticides as a source of indoor air pollution. They are also a source of outdoor air pollution, especially in the form of insect and weed abatement programs.

Many people who know themselves to be susceptible to chemicals move to the suburbs or the countryside to escape from the source of their problem. Having moved to what they think is a safe haven, they are sometimes presented with a worse problem: insect abatement. Sometimes rural or suburban residents are "abated" in the dead of night without any prior warning. Large chemical spraying rigs move through the neighborhood, applying poisons to trees, roadsides, and ponds.

Sleeping quietly in bed with the windows open, a susceptible person's first warning of an abatement rig may be to awake with a strangling cough or even an epilepticlike seizure. I have been called out at night on a number of occasions to resuscitate such people.

Chemically susceptible patients living in areas where these programs exist have to take rather elaborate precautions to guard against such exposures. Some contact the local agencies and ask them for advance notice when their area is to be treated with pesticide sprays. Others flee the area when spraying starts or lock themselves in their homes until the toxic chemicals disperse somewhat.

Yet others attempt to move farther into the country. Sadly, this strategy usually fails, since the abatement programs are often enthusiastically carried out in the rural districts as well. New spraying agencies are continually being formed, or else the escapee runs into trouble with farmers who are spraying for weed and insect control or with foresters spraying their trees. A few of my patients have actually moved back *into the city*, in order to escape the indiscriminate spraying which is now practiced in the countryside!

It is a sad commentary when people must flee to the polluted cities to escape the even worse pollution of the rural areas. Even a drive in the country is now often perilous for chemically susceptible individuals. One may suddenly encounter roadside weed control programs at any time. If this happens, you are well advised to stop, turn the car around, and escape as quickly as possible. An alternative plan is to close the car windows and breathe through an activated carbon filter, if one is available. Even driving along a recently sprayed roadside or railway right-of-way or through a country area immediately after spraying may trigger reactions.[1]

CASE STUDY: CHEMICAL SUSCEPTIBILITY (WEED KILLERS)

In June, 1972, the Johnson family lay sleeping in their rustic house, built along-side a brook in a Western state. At around 6:30 A.M., without prior warning, a helicopter came in low over their rooftop and began discharging a heavy white fog along the power company's right-of-way, which adjoined the house. Four times it swooped down to release a toxic plume of herbicide, in order to kill all vegetation growing beneath the high steel towers of the company.

Although the wind was only three miles per hour that morning, the powerful downdraft of the helicopter's blades propelled the chemicals in the direction of the sleeping household.

Awakened by the sound of the chopper, Mr. Johnson aroused the family, whose members gulped down a hasty breakfast and left the house. As soon as they emerged from the door, however, they were enveloped in a cloud of Tordon 100, a herbicide which contains Pictoran and 2,4-D.

The worst affected was Johnson's teenage daughter, Lydia. She felt nau-seated and dizzy and had persistent headaches for weeks following this incident. Her eyes were dry, with a burning sensation, and she suffered from shortness of breath and coughing, even when the family moved to Johnson's mother's house, miles away. Many bizarre symptoms followed this exposure. All that summer the children were tired almost all the time and slept for long hours at a stretch, although they were normally active and energetic. In Septem-ber, they returned to their home for the first time since the spraying.

The helicopter had left a wide swath of destruction in its path. From the powerlines, over and past their house, and up the hill behind them, the vegetation and plants were either dead, dying, or deformed. A beautiful fig tree which had stood in their yard was leafless and barren.

Not long after this, Johnson was hospitalized with a mysterious "lung problem." By June of the next year, Lydia's eyes no longer focussed properly, and she could not take final exams. Her lips were swollen, and her eyelids were sometimes so enlarged that she could not see out of them. Doctors at a local hospital refused to treat her, however, claiming that her problems were all "psychosomatic" and "hysterical."

By December, 1973, Lydia had trouble walking. She could not maintain her balance and moved in a wobbly fashion, like a drunkard. She had to support herself by hanging onto furniture or clinging to the balustrade when she walked downstairs. Her local general practitioner referred her to a neurologist, who suggested that she was "trying to get attention" by feigning symptoms. He prescribed tranquilizers.

Although not particularly susceptible to chemicals before being "abated," Lydia now became susceptible to many substances, including tobacco smoke, perfumes, deodorants, motor exhausts, gasoline, and so forth. Although her worst symptoms decreased with time, she contracted severe headaches and difficulty in breathing whenever exposed to various chemicals.

When she was tested in my hospital Ecology Unit, she was found to have allergies to wheat, corn, and a number of other foods. More dramatic, however, were her reactions to chemicals commonly encountered in daily life. After having avoided chemical exposure for many days, she was given a feeding of commercial apples, a food which she tolerated in their unsprayed form. The first feeding was followed by repeated clearing of the throat, coughing, and dizziness on sudden change of position. The second feeding of commercial tomato and tomato juice was followed by a sensation of burning in her mouth. A third meal of commercially canned chicken was followed by a headache at ten minutes, which rapidly increased in intensity and was soon accompanied by canker sores in the mouth, aching joints, aching leg muscles, and insomnia that night.

A feeding of commercially canned cherries brought on aching legs, while commercial lettuce caused a stomachache and shaking, quivering, and depression. These symptoms became severe about an hour and a half later, and she also cried and sobbed.

Finally, commercial frozen cauliflower brought on severe depression and crying after fifteen minutes, as well as residual shaking and numbness of the lower limbs on the following morning. It is noteworthy that this numbness was identical in feeling to that which followed the original spraying incident, although it was less severe than that experienced in 1972.

Despite the undemonstrable theories of her neurologists, Lydia Johnson was suffering from the chemical-susceptibility problem, brought on in her case by a massive exposure to herbicide months before. This initial exposure was maintained, albeit at a lower level, by daily exposure to common environmental chemicals, such as residues found in commercial food.

Air pollution from herbicides is becoming more common. Because of the use of similar defoliants during the Vietnam War, some of these effects are becoming better known. One of the chemicals to which Lydia Johnson was exposed, 2,4-D, is also an ingredient in the now infamous Agent Orange. Reports of Vietnam veterans sound remarkably like the symptoms reported by Lydia Johnson. According to one report on such veterans, published in the *New York Times:*

> They say it is a poison that fell from the sky, a herbicide that was supposed to kill only unwanted plants. Instead, they insist, it has made them sick and changed their lives, and even though many years have passed since their exposure to it, they fear it still. They fear it has started processes within them that will make them sick again and perhaps kill them.[2]

No more eloquent—and frightening—condemnation could be made of the virtually unrestrained chemical contamination of our environment.

II
STAGES AND SYMPTOMS OF ENVIRONMENTAL DISEASE

8

Levels of Reaction in Environmental Disease

In the preceding section, the basic concepts of food and chemical susceptibility were presented. In this section, we shall examine how such reactions actually affect patients with a variety of illnesses which are rarely helped by conventional medicine.

The chapters in this section are rather arbitrarily organized around particular diseases. This is, of course, the way conventional medicine, and most patients, think of their ailments. In actuality, however, most susceptible patients have a constellation of diseases, with few clear-cut distinctions between them. The headache patient, if questioned, may turn out to have many localized problems, on the one hand, and a tendency toward depression on the other. Or he may vacillate between periods of exuberance and energy and subsequent "hangovers."

It is the orthodox, overly analytical medical system which insists on pigeon-holing patients into disease categories, and, particularly, separating physical from "mental" or "emotional" problems. Whatever the practical benefits of such a scheme, it fails to describe these various complaints as part of an overall continuum of ill-health in the life of each individual patient.

What is meant by "headache" or "arthritis" below, then, is a stage of illness in which arthritis or headache is the *principal*, but rarely the sole, complaint. These levels of reaction were first described in 1956.[1]

The bulk of the cases presented here fall either into the plus-two, the minus-two, or the minus-three categories. In other words, they are intermediate between the least and the most extreme cases of both stimulation and withdrawal. The reasons for my emphasis on these conditions are as follows.

STIMULATORY LEVELS

Plus-one cases are rarely seen by a physician. The plus-one patient is basically a happy person, mildly stimulated by a "natural high." He rarely, if ever, thinks of himself as a candidate for serious illness.

Plus-three and plus-four cases, on the other hand, are sometimes brought to a physician, and such cases could be presented. (In her manic phase, for instance, Nora Barnes was a plus-four case.) These cases are relatively rare, however, since before the average food or chemical addict reaches this stage, his withdrawal symptoms have usually become more and more pronounced. It is this withdrawal phase which brings him to the doctor's office—not the previous "high."

This is why a discussion of stimulatory reactions focuses on the plus-two stage. It is here that we find at least three serious medical problems: hyperactivity in both children and adults; obesity; and alcoholism, the acme of the food-addiction problem.

WITHDRAWAL LEVELS

Minus-one Levels. As was explained earlier, there are four progressive levels of withdrawal. Of these, the localized symptoms of the minus-one level are certainly the best known and probably the most common. Of the various organ systems involved with localized allergies, the upper respiratory tract (nose, sinuses, and throat) probably is most frequently affected. For instance, the practices of ear, nose, and throat physicians as well as many allergists are dominated by seasonal (hay fever) and perennial nasal allergy. The lower respiratory complaints of coughing (bronchitis) and wheezing (bronchial asthma and its complications) are also very common. Although these minus-one reactions most often occur in response to such inhaled particles as pollens, dust, mold spores, animal danders, or debris from insects, they may also be caused by food or environmental chemicals.

Minus-one localized allergic reactions involving the gastrointestinal and genitourinary systems, also of common occurrence, are most frequently responses to foods and environmental chemical exposures. Allergic skin manifestations are of two types. Direct contact reactions usually result from exposure to chemicals in the environment. Eczema from ingested exposures is usually caused by foods or food additives.

From the standpoint of their recognition and management, reactions to inhaled particles (pollens, dusts, molds, and so forth) are far better handled by orthodox medical treatment than those caused by exposure to foods and environmental chemicals. Since these localized allergies are described adequately in most other books on allergy, they will not be emphasized in this presentation, although it should be restated that most cases of hay fever and other local allergies can be benefitted by the methods outlined here.

Minus-two Levels. Minus-two reactions are *systemic*, or more generalized, reactions. These will be emphasized in this book both because of their common occurrence and because their environmental causes—especially common foods and chemical exposures—are so rarely recognized. The major manifestations are fatigue and pain, especially headache, and muscle and joint aches and pains.

Minus-three and Minus-four Levels. In contrast to minus-one and minus-two withdrawal levels characterized by physical symptoms, minus-three and minus-four levels are concerned with mental and behavioral responses. Minus-three, called "brain-fag," is characterized by mental confusion and relatively less severe depression. Complaints in this category are most commonly regarded as psychological and are rarely handled from the standpoint of their environmental origin. This brain-fag level will be emphasized with case histories.

Minus-four reactions include the most severe forms of depression. These cerebral and behavioral reactions, usually referred to as psychoses, may be characterized by abnormalities of perception and consciousness. Although such extreme cases may also be helped by the application of the techniques of clinical ecology, since I am an internist I see relatively fewer cases at this level than do psychiatrists. Despite the demonstrable relationships between many "mental" problems and allergic reactions, ecologically oriented techniques are applied with greater difficulty to longstanding and advanced cases of psychosis, especially schizophrenia, than to less advanced cases.

Before discussing specific cases, however, it may be worthwhile to review briefly the kinds of problems which can be caused by the stimulatory and withdrawal reactions. This will give some idea of the scope of these disorders and the position of specific symptoms in the overall scheme.

Plus-one reactions are usually within the range of normal behavior. The person in this stage is slightly overactive but tends to be relatively happy and symptom-free.

Plus-two reactions include hyperactivity, irritability, excessive hunger and thirst; insomnia; restlessness; nervousness, jitteriness, overresponsiveness, negativism; shortened attention span and learning disorders; vasomotor changes, such as chilling, flushing, and sweating; obesity, alcoholism, and drug addiction.

Plus-three reactions include egocentrism; drunklike behavior, with muscular incoordination; sensations of floating and unreality; anxiety and extreme nervousness; extreme apprehension and fearfulness.

Plus-four reactions include mania, with or without convulsions; epileptic or catatonic seizures; muscle-twitching, jerking of extremities; frenzy, aggression, agitation, panic; repetitive thinking, speech, and actions. (The word "mania" is used according to common, rather than psychiatric, usage.)

Patients may have only one of these symptoms. More commonly, however, they suffer from a number of different problems. They may straddle several of these categories by being, say, nervous and jittery $(++)$ at one time and egocentric and anxious at another $(+++)$. Or they may vacillate between one of these stimulatory levels and a more or less corresponding withdrawal level.

Some of the more common forms of stimulatory reactions are given in the chapters which follow. Although hyperactivity and alcoholism will be described, chapters have not been written on the subjects of obesity and drug addiction because of space limitations.

Suffice it to say, briefly, that obesity and alcoholism are basically similar illnesses, one dealing with addicting foods in their edible form and the other in their potable form. Stimulatory phases in both instances tend to be relatively prolonged, inasmuch as victims tend to be aware of the general nature of the responsible addictants in both instances, although specific addictants may not be pinpointed. This seems to be especially true in obesity, which is more often related to eating in general than to the frequent use of one or more specific foods. Although there is some habituation involved, cravings in obesity can usually be curbed effectively as a result of the avoidance of incriminated foods.

The basic course of addictive illness is shown in Figure 1. It is believed to start with food addiction, as shown at the base of this pyramid with food fractions listed in the ascending order of their relative speed of absorption (fats and oils, proteins, starches, sugars and alcohols).

From this base, addictive responses to food-drug combinations and drugs commonly occur, as addicted persons tend to seek ever more effective stimulatory effects. Heroin, administered by intravenous injection, has long been known as the apex of addictive phenomena.

Patients may be seen at any stage of this process, involving various combinations of addictants.

9
Hyperactivity (Plus-two Reaction)

One of the major forms of plus-two reactions is hyperactivity. This is also sometimes called hyperkinesis. Far more common in males than females, it is marked by distractability, inappropriate responses, and irritability.[1] Supercharged and jittery behavior can occur at any age but is particularly common among children. It is often accompanied by aggressive actions, temper tantrums, poor schoolwork, and sometimes by overweight. This was first described in 1947.[2]

This sort of behavior has become increasingly common among children, and many theories have been advanced to account for it, ranging from Freudian interpretations of family life to the incrimination of television violence. Often, however, the problem is an allergic/addictive response to some food eaten in a compulsive fashion or to some chemical encountered in the course of everyday life. Removal of these substances and overall environmental control can often help such children in a dramatic way.

CASE STUDY: HYPERACTIVITY WITH TEMPER TANTRUMS

Barry Carter was a terror. At eight years of age, he had been a difficult child for as long as his parents could remember. For years he had thrown temper tantrums whenever he could not get his way, but when the family moved into a new house he became increasingly tired, listless, and irritable. When Barry started school that September, all his problems came to the fore. After three miserable months in school, at home, and in the neighborhood, Barry was brought to me.

That winter, Barry had gotten into the habit of kicking his mother in the shins and placing all responsibility for his problems on the poor woman. He terrorized and beat up his younger "playmates" both at school and on the street. The principal and other school officials declared that he not only was unteachable, but that his irritability, hyperactivity, and uncontrolled behavior disturbed the entire class. The school urged the parents to remove Barry from school and take him to a psychiatrist. Their theory was that Mrs. Carter had "rejected and dejected" her son. He was put on Ritalin, a drug often used to treat hyperactivity.

The parents had tried this psychiatric route; they also had tried spanking him repeatedly. Nothing seemed to work.

Several interesting facts emerged from his history. One tell-tale clue was that Barry's symptoms were always *accentuated in winter*. In particular, he had become increasingly disrespectful, hostile, and sassy since the beginning of the heating season. This suggested a chemical cause—particularly, something connected to the home heating system. Upon learning that an auxiliary gas-fired space heater had been installed in his bedroom the previous summer, it was recommended that he exchange rooms with his older sister. Although his behavior improved, he still remained too hyperactive and distraught to read with any comprehension.

By this point, the child and his mother were not even talking to each other. An experiment was tried, to see how the child would react to a new environment. He went with his grandmother, to stay in a hotel room, which was free of those environmental chemicals which frequently cause or perpetuate chronic symptoms.

Within the first three days of fasting, drinking only spring water, and taking no drugs, Barry's pulse decreased from 90 to 70 (an increased pulse is often a sign of allergic reactions [Chap. 16]). Barry now read incessantly, the first time he had been able to do so in months. After completing a battery of food allergy tests, he returned to his home city, on good terms with his mother. Upon returning to school directly from the hotel, he apologized for his past behavior and asked for makeup work. However, that afternoon upon returning home for the first time, he developed a headache. By the following morning he was tired, listless, pale, and puffy around the eyes, and within three days had returned to his previous level. For example, upon arising he ripped his favorite Boy Scout uniform to shreds, kicked the baby, and attacked his mother.

His parents removed the gas space-heater from his room but did not change the gas-fired hot-air system which heated the entire house. Thus, although his symptoms improved greatly that summer, they were back in full force when the heat was turned on again in the fall.

Changing the gas-fired system for an all-electric heating and cooking system brought about a complete change in Barry's behavior. His hyperactive, irritable, and destructive traits disappeared. He remained quite well, only suffering relapses when exposed to other sources of gas outside the home, or to heavy smog or pollution.

He was suffering from the chemical-susceptibility problem, which was mainly exhibited as a plus-two hyperactive reaction to environmental chemicals, particularly gas.

CASE STUDY: HYPERACTIVITY WITH FOOD ALLERGY

A similar case was that of Ralph Hodgson, a twelve-year-old, prone to temper tantrums and hyperactive behavior. He had been having tantrums since the age of one. He had been to a number of psychiatrists for treatment. Since Ralph had an older brother and a younger sister, both of whom were model children, the psychiatrist attributed Ralph's problem to the fact that he was a middle child, contending that middle children were more prone to such behavior.

Ralph was repeatedly caught lying and stealing. He frequently beat the family dog and succeeded in killing one pet gerbil and mutilating another. He built model planes but only, it seemed, to have the pleasure of smashing them. He also broke several chairs and damaged the furniture.

His I.Q. was above average, and all the standard physical and psychological tests revealed no organic problem. Yet he had great difficulty sleeping and could only sleep at times with the motor of a hair drier running near his bed. (The reason for this quirk was never explained.) If another family member entered his room, he ordered him out. The final straw for his parents was when they returned from a party and found a distraught baby sitter sobbing in the living room. Ralph had pounded a hole in the plaster wall between his bedroom and the living room and was climbing in and out.

Since Ralph's mother suffered from ecologic illness of her own, I suggested that both she and the boy be hospitalized together. In this way they could help each other and observe one another's progress. There was a bit of self-interest in this, too, since I knew that it would be extremely difficult to care for a wild twelve-year-old for three weeks in a closed hospital ward. I call this joint treatment of several family members "observed togetherness."[2]

The boy's medical history suggested that he might have food allergies. For instance, he was tremendously fond of orange juice, preferring it over any other beverage. He loved hard candy (which is almost pure corn sugar). His mother, Lorraine, age forty-one, had been subject to rheumatoid arthritis involving the elbows, knees, ankles, hips, and back for the previous eight years. She had also had sinus symptoms, headaches, and chronic fatigue, on and off, for years.

The program employed in my Ecology Unit will be described in greater detail in Chapter 17. Basically, the patient fasts for five days and then is allowed to test one food after another in a search for definitive reactions. One of the first foods Ralph was tested on was orange juice, because of his addictivelike craving for it. At first he seemed normal, but within about two hours he was flushed in the face, had started to pack his bags, and insulted his mother and the staff. When his father told him, over the phone, that he could not come home, he hung up on him. Ralph struck his mother twice before his father and I arrived on the scene simultaneously. The room was completely disheveled. When I suggested that the oranges were the cause of this reaction, he started screaming and tore his symptom chart to shreds.

A few days later he had a similar but less severe reaction to grapefruit, another member of the citrus family. He also had less troublesome reactions to pork, peanuts, corn, peas, and bananas. Once all of these foods were scrupulously avoided, Ralph's behavior improved greatly. When I last saw him, he was doing fine and had developed an excellent insight into his problem. His schoolwork and interpersonal relationships were now generally excellent.

An interesting side note concerns Mrs. Hodgson. As she went through the food tests, she discovered that a number of frequently eaten foods—including carrots, rice, pork, halibut, oranges, wheat, corn, peas, and grapefruit—caused acute flare-ups of her arthritic pain. By avoiding these foods and then rotating her diet according to the rules that I shall explain, she reaped equal benefit from her stay in the Ecology Unit.

The case of Ralph Hodgson illustrates the role of food addiction in causing the plus-two reaction of hyperactivity. The fact that he and his mother were both helped at the same time shows that sometimes problems which appear to be entirely "emotional" turn out to be environmental.

When two family members have been at each other's throats, it is sometimes advantageous to hospitalize them both at the same time. In this way they see that it is not their personalities which are at fault, but that a physical problem lies at the base of their difficulties.

CASE STUDY: HYPERACTIVITY WITH AUTISM

The previous two cases illustrated a chemical- and a food-susceptibility problem, respectively. The case of ten-year-old Paul Rossi demonstrates the more common instance in which both food and chemical susceptibilities combine to create a serious illness.

Paul was an extreme case of hyperactivity. The examining physician in the Ecology Unit could not complete the admission interview, since Paul kicked, pushed, and shoved everybody around him, including his mother who was to stay with him.

Paul's temper tantrums had begun when he was thirteen months old. He appeared to be learning well, however, until his seventeenth month, when he suddenly started forgetting the words he had already learned. He seemed distant and unable to relate emotionally to those around him. When he reached school age, his parents attempted to place him in a public school, but to no avail. He could not learn, and was transferred from one school to another. He was finally placed in a school for problem children, a sheltered environment, where he was kept on tranquilizers most of the time. Occasionally his behavior became so uncontrollable that he had to be placed in a straitjacket.

Watching this boy race around the examination room, overturning furniture and tearing papers, one could not help but feel sorry for this tortured child and his frustrated, agonized parents.

Paul had been diagnosed as "autistic." Autism is a strange disease in which the child, in effect, dreams his life away, seemingly unaware of external reality. He cannot form meaningful relationships, and has difficulty in learning or even speaking. Other doctors had suggested as treatment drugs, vitamins, or institutionalization. Before coming to the Ecology Unit, Mrs. Rossi had put Paul on the Feingold Diet, a mass-applicable approach which cautions against artificially-colored or -flavored items, as well as certain other types of food.[3] The Feingold Diet, which eliminates *some*, but hardly all, of the synthetic pollutants in food, was useful, and Paul benefitted. Encouraged, Mrs. Rossi sought a more complete, personalized approach.

Paul's history revealed a tendency toward addiction to foods containing beet sugar, milk, corn, and oranges. These seemed to result in flare-ups of his behavior problems when he ate them in excess. He also appeared to be highly susceptible to environmental chemicals. When he was exposed to perfume, nail polish, or similar cosmetics he would frequently scream, kick, and bite for a few minutes, as if in a seizure.

Abstention from food for five days, in a chemically less contaminated environment, led to a marked improvement in his behavior. When he was given beef, and corn mush sprinkled with corn sugar, however, he threw a temper tantrum which was quite convincing as a test of food allergy to those around him. He also reacted to apricot, raisins, grape juice, yeast, beets and beet sugar, honey, lamb, and other foods. His mother had said that hot dogs seemed to bring on his symptoms at home. Most hot dogs contain beef, corn, and other foods identified as troublesome in the deliberate food tests.

We next took some of the organic foods to which Paul had not reacted in his food tests (such as honeydew, broccoli, and peas) and fed them to him for six successive meals in their commercial form—the type of food that he, and millions of other children and adults, eat every day. By the end of the sixth meal, there was a marked increase in his hyperactivity and irritability, and the symptoms of autism were also increased.

Paul turned out to be one of those people who must have truly organic food in order to stay well. If he does not get it he suffers from problems so severe that he becomes impossible for his parents to cope with. With it, despite the supposedly "incurable" nature of his problems, specifically autism, he is able to lead a normal life.

CASE STUDY: BEHAVIOR PROBLEMS, HEARING LOSS, AND HYPERACTIVITY

David Hart was eight years old when he was brought to me. His problems were obvious: his face was never at peace, but was wracked by spasms; he was continually sniffing, blinking, and squinting. His eyes were red and rimmed by dark circles. Although his grades were average, he had frequent temper tantrums at school and at home.

In addition, David had a hearing problem, which seemed to increase as he grew older. He complained of a ringing in his ears, a condition called tinnitus. This had been unsuccessfully treated with decongestants and antihistamines. Sometimes he complained of having a "bug in his ear." The slightest noise in class distracted him, since then he could no longer hear the teacher distinctly.

The routine five-day water fast in the Ecology Unit worked wonders: the mouth tic, eye-blinking, and hyperactivity disappeared. So, too, did the bags under the eyes, which are called "allergic shiners," a frequent sign of food or chemical susceptibility.

When single foods, known not to have been significantly contaminated with chemicals, were returned to David's diet, some of them brought on attacks of spasms and facial contortions. The worst offenders in his case were wheat, beef, corn, and blueberries, followed by haddock, cherries, peanuts, and potatoes.

Many foods, however, could be eaten without causing any symptoms, such as crab, chicken, pork, lamb, and onion. When some of these acceptable foods were given to David in their commercial, supermarket form, however, they caused grimaces, hyperactivity, eye circles, and gassiness. The boy became progressively more grouchy and twitchy after the second feeding of "normal" food, and this increased with each subsequent feeding. The avoidance of such foods paved the way for David's recovery, and the last time I spoke to his family, he was greatly improved and doing well in school.

Like Paul Rossi, David was one of those hyperactive children whose problem was actually caused by a highly individualized reaction to the food and chemical environment, and greatly helped by avoiding those items to which he was allergic.

CASE STUDY: HEADACHE, STOMACHACHE, AND ALLERGIC BRAIN REACTION

A slightly different kind of problem was presented by Karen Black. She complained, not just of hyperactivity and restlessness, but of headaches, stomachaches, skin rash, and a peculiar "spaced out" feeling in her head much of the time.

Her history provided a good clue: the symptoms became much worse after the family had moved so that she had to travel for a long time to get back and forth from school. In retrospect, this may have been due to an increased exposure to exhaust fumes. She developed stomachaches and an itchy rash under her armpits. A perceptive doctor advised her to stop wearing synthetic garments, and the rash went away, but the stomach problem and other symptoms persisted.

The family moved again, and now Karen developed a headache whenever she rode in the family car. Her teachers complained that she was in a world of her own, and before the end of the fifth grade the family had to remove her from school entirely and seek home instruction for her.

Because there was a strong family history of allergies, Karen was taken to a clinical ecologist. He diagnosed her as allergic to a variety of foods, including apple, chicken, grape, milk, peanuts, and rice, all of which made her feel "spaced out" on the provocative test (see Chap. 16).

To get a more definitive answer, Karen was referred to me. Upon fasting, she underwent withdrawal symptoms which, as I shall explain more fully below, are typical for those suffering from this syndrome. On the fourth day of the water fast, she felt sick to her stomach and threw up. Soon, however, she felt better—better, in fact, than she had in a long time.

Deliberate test feedings revealed a very serious allergy to cane, chicken, peanuts, corn, grapes and raisins, beef, milk, wheat, lobster, and peas, and lesser reactions to lamb, yeast, apples, and cherries.

Eating these foods would bring on her old symptoms, including periods of anger or tiredness. She complained of being "spacey" and "down," although this alternated with irritable periods.

Smelling chemicals made her angry, tired, dull, and almost catatonic. Two consecutive meals of commercial foods contaminated with the "normal" amounts of chemicals made her tired, irritable, with episodes of staring vacantly into space.

The testing was quite successful, and Karen was like a new person upon leaving the hospital. Unfortunately, she went back into a house which was ecologically harmful for her. It had brand new carpeting with a foam rubber pad, both of which are often the source of adverse reactions among those with the chemical-susceptibility problem. What is more, the family's furniture had been put into storage several months before and appeared to have been fumigated—a common practice among storage companies. All of these factors combined to make Karen's recovery less complete than it could have been.

Hyperactivity and related syndromes are a growing problem in the United States. Rather than dealing with this problem at the level of environmental *causation*, orthodox medicine prefers to perpetuate the problem through the use of drugs. Of the 750,000 children seen for "minimal brain dysfunction" (another term for hyperactivity) in 1978, 212,000 were put on medication, and about 75 percent of them, or nearly 120,000 on methylphenidate hydrochloride (Ritalin Hydrochloride).[4]

A child psychologist recently complained that labeling a hyperactive child as in need of drugs eliminates the necessity of discovering the underlying problem which is causing his behavior problems. While the psychologist probably had in mind psychological causes, the same can be said, even more emphatically, about the chemical and environmental causes of this disorder.[5]

10
Alcoholism (Plus-two Reaction)

We are so imbued with psychological explanations of alcoholism that it seems strange to consider this problem as related to food or chemical susceptibility. Frequently, however, an alcoholic is not a mentally sick person, in the conventional sense, but a very advanced food addict. In fact, alcoholism could well be called the acme, or pinnacle, of the food-addiction pyramid.

It is usually assumed that the alcoholic craves the ethyl alcohol in his drink. In most discussions of the problem, however, a significant fact is overlooked: few people would choose to drink pure ethyl alcohol, even if given the chance. Alcohol is almost invariably found mixed with other ingredients or fractions, many of them related to common foods. Starting in the mid-1940s, I began to accumulate evidence that it was principally these foods, rather than the alcohol itself, to which many alcoholics were addicted.

This insight was related to developments in food allergy. It was Herbert J. Rinkel, the same man who discovered "masking" and "unmasking" of food allergy (Chap. 1), who first diagnosed allergies to corn, in the 1940s. I confirmed Rinkel's observations in my patients, and together we published a series of lists of foods containing corn or corn products.

Allergy to corn turned out to be the most common food allergy in North America. Why, then, had its discovery waited until the 1940s, years after the other common allergies were described? The answer lay in the very fact of corn's popularity. Because it was present in practically every meal in one form or another, obvious or disguised, it was extremely difficult to unmask. It was only when we had compiled a fairly complete list and ferreted out the corn in numerous products, in the form of corn syrup, corn starch, corn oil, and so forth, that we could perform adequate tests.

Soon after this, I began to notice that many of my alcoholic patients had corn allergies. Some patients, for example, told me that they became drunk on only one or two glasses of beer or a couple of shots of bourbon. Such patients were invariably highly susceptible to corn or to other *ingredients* in these beverages, such as wheat or yeast. It dawned on me that it might be these substances, rather than the alcohol per se, which perpetuated the craving for alcoholic beverages and which caused the bizarre behavioral changes associated with alcohol consumption. Since alcohol is rapidly absorbed into the bloodstream, it was likely that these food fractions were rapidly absorbed along with it, creating problems for the susceptible.

CASE STUDY: ALCOHOLISM AND FOOD ALLERGY

This theory was confirmed in the case of Ted Parsons, whom I first saw in 1948. Parsons had been a successful executive, on the way up, associated with a large company in Chicago. After a rapid rise he had become, over a period of years, an alcoholic. He was suspended from his job and actually became a "skid row" type of drunkard.

With his family's help, he had managed to pull out of this nosedive and had become a founding member of the Alcoholics Anonymous group in his area. But after ten years "on the wagon," he had begun to backslide. Another interval of alcoholism ensued, followed by a period of abstinence. This time, however, he recovered his sobriety but not his health. When he was not drinking, he suffered from extreme fatigue and almost constant headaches.

In preparing to perform food-ingestion tests with corn and wheat (which from an allergy point of view is virtually identical to barley and malt), he avoided these foods for four days. His fatigue was greatly accentuated for two days as a withdrawal reaction, following which he felt much better. During the test with wheat porridge, he developed progressive nasal obstruction and fatigue, as well as tautness of the nape of his neck and delayed dizziness. Reactions persisted for several days.

Some nasal symptoms and fatigue were still present prior to Parsons' corn test four days later. The trial ingestion of corn porridge and corn sugar was also followed by a progressive increase in fatigue and some staggering upon leaving the office. Fearing that he might head for the nearest bar on the way home, I placed him in a taxi, paid the driver to take him home directly, and called his wife to tell her what I had done. His fatigue increased during the night.

Parsons called me the next morning and commented, "It is funny to have a hangover twenty-one months after having stopped drinking. There is no difference between the fatigue this morning and a bad alcoholic hangover." He went on to describe how he had to crawl to the bathroom because he was too weak and dizzy to walk, but that his lassitude, dizziness, and uneasiness could be relieved just like that (as if by a snap of the fingers) with a drink.

When he asked, "What is wrong with me?" I explained that he was having a true hangover—not from bourbon, but from corn, its principal ingredient. He had apparently been allergic to wheat (barley malt) and corn, as well as certain other foods, for years without realizing it. His addiction to bourbon had been an attempt to get a high level of cereal grains into his system as rapidly as possible and to maintain that level of stimulation. His more recent headache and fatigue could be explained by the perpetuation of his corn and wheat (barley malt) addictions, but at a much lower, unsatisfactory level, by the use of more slowly absorbed wheat- and corn-containing foods.

By the avoidance of wheat, corn, and a few other incriminated foods, Parsons' headache and fatigue not only subsided, but what is more, his craving for alcohol disappeared.

This craving is, of course, the bane of many ex-alcoholics' existence. One can, with extraordinary willpower, stop drinking, but it is far harder to conquer the desire to drink. Parsons' case suggested a possible reason for this. The consumption of other grain-containing foods would perpetuate the underlying problem—food addiction/allergy. Thus, in a sense, the alcoholic is never completely free of his "alcoholism" as long as he is consuming the foods which constitute his addictant.

Parsons, for instance, carried around with him a pocket full of candies containing corn sugar, which he sucked whenever he had the urge to drink. This was, in fact, the standard operating procedure of his Alcoholics Anonymous unit. Through practice, these individuals had found that they could relieve their craving for grain-containing alcoholic beverages by sucking on another rapidly absorbed form of grain. They had, in effect, transferred food addiction in its highest form—alcoholism—to food addiction in a less severe (and from the addict's point of view, less satisfactory) form, corn sugar addiction. When Parsons realized that he was actually *perpetuating* his problem by eating this candy, he stopped immediately and avoided all contact with wheat, corn, and related foods which had been implicated.

It was through Parsons that I became acquainted with the members of Alcoholics Anonymous in the Chicago area. In the late 1940s, I carried out a study of forty-four members of this organization. I attended meetings, but instead of participating in discussions (which was forbidden to outsiders, under the organization's rules), I stayed in the kitchen and interviewed members. Their histories, at least, suggested a strong correlation between alcoholism and susceptibility to the various food components of alcoholic beverages.

What are these food components? It soon became apparent that the study of alcoholism from the point of view of clinical ecology was hampered by the lack of information on the manufacture of liquor. Through much detective work, it was possible to track down the components of various drinks, though some of this information was guarded as trade secrets. Government regulation in this respect was lax, and alcohol was not regulated by the Food and Drug Administration but by the less food-conscious Treasury Department.

Gradually it was possible to put together a comprehensive theory of alcoholism as the apex of food allergy (the term "food addiction" did not come into use until 1952). According to this view, alcoholism is the acme of the food-allergy problem because alcohol is rapidly absorbed all along the gastrointestinal tract, from the mouth to the stomach to the intestines. Food, on the other hand, is mainly absorbed in the intestines, and more slowly at that.

There were four facts about alcohol which did not seem to fit into the theory. Their existence threw doubt on the entire concept. Wanting to obtain pure samples of corn mash whiskey, and other pure items for testing, I called a meeting with the research and technical directors of a major Illinois distillery. I presented my theory to them and pointed out the four existing discrepancies:

1. Why did corn-sensitive patients react to Scotch whiskey? Scotch comes from the British Isles but no corn (maize) grows there.
2. Why did grape-sensitive patients react to Puerto Rican and Cuban rum but not to Jamaican rum?
3. Why did corn-sensitive patients also react to apple brandy? The public relations officer of the producer of the brand in question had assured me that no corn went into the manufacture of their product.
4. Why did corn-sensitive patients react adversely to a popular American brandy but not to French brandy?

The research and technical directors of this distillery had been polite but somewhat skeptical, when I first presented this possible interpretation of alcoholism. But as I explained apparent exceptions to the theory, they became increasingly interested. They not only knew some of the answers but began to fill in some of the holes in the theory themselves.

First, all-malt Scotch whiskey is made of dried, roasted barley or malt, which, from the allergy standpoint, is closely related to wheat, if not virtually identical with it. But blended Scotch whiskey manufactured for export to the United States is blended with cereal-grain whiskey made from corn which is shipped from the United States or Argentina. Thus, persons sensitive to corn could be expected to react to it.

Second, Jamaican rum, like other rums, is made from cane. However, the laws of Jamaica demand that rum manufactured there be bottled on the island, whereas Cuban and Puerto Rican rums are shipped from their home ports to the United States in big hogshead barrels. Most of these were then blended with up to two-and-one-half percent grape brandy before bottling. Hence, grape-sensitive patients could be expected to react to the Cuban and Puerto Rican rums.

The distillery experts were not sure why the patients sensitive to corn reacted to apple brandy, however, and the whole theory was put in doubt when the manufacturer told me that the product did not contain corn. But after testing a few more patients highly sensitive to corn and confirming my earlier impression, I wrote the president of the company manufacturing this brand of apple brandy and suggested that the person answering my earlier inquiry had misled me. In the meantime, I had learned about trade practices in the liquor industry and asked specifically what the source of the caramel was which was used to maintain uniformity of color in the brandy. No one knew, off-hand. But upon corresponding with the manufacturer of this product, they learned that it was made from half corn sugar (dextrose) and half cane sugar.

Fourth, the possible corn content of the popular brand of grape brandy which precipitated reactions in corn-sensitive patients could not be confirmed through correspondence with the manufacturer of the product. But upon visiting their California plant in the early 1950s, I learned that corn sugar was used in its production.

This interpretation of alcoholism has not been widely accepted, either by those responsible for the policies of Alcoholics Anonymous or by those who teach courses on alcoholism. One apparent reason is that many alcoholics were quick to grasp an implication of this theory: namely, that some reformed alcoholics could drink compatible alcoholic beverages as long as they avoided both drinks and foods prepared from those substances to which they were allergic. In other words, a corn-sensitive patient who was a confirmed bourbon alcoholic could drink some wines and rums, provided these alcoholic beverages were free of cereal grains and he was not susceptible to grape, cane, or yeast. The effects of alcohol per se on the body did not seem to be an appreciable cause of alcoholism.

It should be emphasized, however, that the prospect of social drinking of compatible alcoholic beverages is not for all alcoholics. Although such a program may be possible for an alcoholic having a very limited food allergy problem, it cannot be considered if one is yeast-sensitive, because yeast is present in all alcoholic beverages. Also, the person who already has a wide base of food allergy usually also has a tendency to develop new food allergies readily, even though he indulges in a compatible alcoholic beverage in moderate amounts and only once, or at the most, twice, weekly. Not only the foods used in manufacturing an alcoholic beverage but also the foods eaten while drinking must be taken into account, due to the extremely rapid absorption of food-alcohol mixtures. In order to minimize the chance of sensitivity spreading to other items of the diet, *all* compatible foods—including those entering food-alcohol mixtures—should be used according to the principles of the Rotary Diversified Diet (see Chap. 18).

The only way to know whether one is actually sensitive to corn, wheat (rye, barley, malt), or other grains, yeast, grape, potato, or other ingredients of alcoholic beverages is to undergo extensive food testing. And only in the presence of a food allergy problem of limited extent (a distinct minority of cases) should social drinking of compatible alcoholic beverages by reformed alcoholics be considered.

In the great bulk of addicted drinkers of alcoholic beverages, abstinence from drinking, according to the Alcoholics Anonymous approach, is still the most highly successful rehabilitation program. However, there are obstacles in the application of this program, because this concept of alcoholism is not widely known.

My interpretation of alcoholism was first published in various medical journals starting in 1950.[1,2] This view has also been confirmed by several clinical ecologists, including Richard Mackarness of England and Marshall Mandell of this country.[3,4] My list of the food sources entering the manufacturing of alcoholic beverages has been published recently.[5]

CASE HISTORY: ALCOHOLISM, ANXIETY, AND MENTAL DISORIENTATION

Diane Witherspoon was in her early forties and had started having a problem with alcohol when she worked as a stewardess, more than a decade before. Her excessive drinking continued when she got an influential job in politics and became exacerbated when she got married and had a child. Within three days of giving birth, in fact, she got drunk, and, she says, remained intoxicated for most of the next three years.

This period of alcoholism was preceded, during her pregnancy, by a craving for sweets and a weight gain of sixty pounds.

During her three-year period of alcoholism, she drank a fifth of vodka a day. At times she became so nervous that she shook violently. The only way that she could relieve this shaking was to drink more vodka. She could no longer read, since she had "floaters" in the form of dots, threads, beads, and circles drifting across her field of vision. On one occasion, while bathing her child, she was overcome with uncontrollable rage at some meaningless remark and violently beat the youngster.

After living as a virtual recluse, she managed to drag herself to a local church and appeal to the minister for help. He referred her to Alcoholics Anonymous. AA exhorted her to abandon drink.

None of this seemed to help. She still had "cobwebs" in her head, nervousness, fits of anxiety, visual distortions, and "floaters." And she still had a craving for alcoholic beverages.

Mrs. Witherspoon drank tea compulsively and began to suspect that it was not agreeing with her. She suspected the sugar she added to the tea, and so she eliminated it, with no beneficial effect. She then tried other beverages, such as herb tea and even plain hot water. Everything seemed to make her feel worse. Her psychiatrist predictably accused her of being "neurotic" about food. (It was not until she came to the Ecology Unit that she discovered that she was sensitive to all *chlorinated* water.)

A perceptive woman, she began to find clues of her food susceptibilities, although she had never heard of clinical ecology. After eating a salami sandwich once, she felt as if she were about to explode from nervousness. She waited a few days and then experimented by trying salami again. Again she experienced a nervous attack. She did this four times.

Having learned about clinical ecology through a lecture, she was admitted to the Ecology Unit. In her initial interview, she cried constantly and was in a state of nervous exhaustion. After a few days of fasting on pure water, however, she was symptom-free and almost euphoric. When she began to test various waters, in sequence, she had a serious reaction to one particular water. It turned out to be from Lake Michigan sources, the same kind she drank at home and out of which she had made her tea.

Upon testing she was found to have some degree of susceptibility to almost every food tested. We call such persons "universal reactors," and they have a serious problem indeed. On her second morning, she was given pears for breakfast. "My mind closed down," she later recalled, "and my brain was floating around as if on water. There was no way to lock it into place. I could not talk or converse. I could hear words coming out of peoples' mouths, but I could not respond."

Usually, but not always, one reacts most strongly to those foods which one eats regularly, more than once every three days. Pears were not listed among such foods in her history. Upon further inquiry, it turned out that she had had a pear tree in her backyard as a child and had eaten them compulsively and to excess at that time. It is entirely possible that this early, excessive exposure had left her with a fixed allergy to the fruit.

Her most dramatic reaction was to potato. She had finished her first boiled potato and was eating her second when, five minutes or so into the test, she crumpled over in agony. She later said that the pain was the worst she had ever experienced in her life, worse than her difficult childbirth.

When she left the hospital, Mrs. Witherspoon's prescription was to avoid those foods to which she had the strongest reactions, try to find new, compatible foods, and eventually try to reintroduce some of her "failed" foods back into her diet. In her case, however, all alcoholic beverages were taboo, because she was susceptible to various components of all of them.

To summarize, the treatment of alcoholism by the methods of clinical ecology has been successful in many cases. It even has been possible to permit some alcoholic beverages, in limited amounts, to former alcoholics, provided they only take compatible beverages, in a rotated schedule. Whether this can be done depends on the individual nature of the case.

Alcoholics, like schizophrenics, need a supportive atmosphere in which to recover. If the family unit is still intact, the patient frequently does very well. But an alcoholic who has no family, and who eats in restaurants frequently, has a much smaller chance of making a full recovery through the methods of clinical ecology. The reason is that most American alcoholics are highly corn-sensitive, and there is some form of corn in almost every commercially prepared meal.

In order to go on this program, then, the reformed alcoholic must either make his own meals, according to his individual needs (as determined by food tests), or have someone with the necessary knowledge to prepare them for him. In practice, these needs could best be met inside a functioning family unit. The homeless alcoholic is likely to leave the Ecology Unit in decent shape, go out to eat, and immediately resume his addiction to corn, wheat, or whatever was making him sick in the first place. This "up" phase may last an hour or two, as in the case of Mr. Parsons, before he starts to come down and experience a kind of "hangover." The experienced alcoholic, however, knows very well how to ward off a hangover—and before long he is in a bar, drinking down his dose of corn or wheat in convenient liquid form.

Similarly, an alcoholic who has not worked out his food allergies along the lines indicated in this book has little chance of breaking the addiction for good, since he is constantly being restimulated by contact with the very foods which lie at the basis of his problem. It is as if a heroin addict were given a small amount of his craved substance just as he was trying to get over his addiction. Yet the alcoholic is unaware of the real nature of his craving and takes the wrong substance unintentionally. He is left with a constant craving for alcoholic beverages and must exercise extraordinary willpower to fight off his physiological need.

The safest course for anyone who fears alcoholism is not to drink more often than once every four days and only to drink those beverages (or eat those foods) to which he knows that he is not allergic.

11
Withdrawal Levels of Reaction

A food or chemical susceptibility usually starts with an addictive type of response, a "high" reaction. In time, however, this usually gives way to increasing periods of illness or depression. Sooner or later, the "down" phases become predominant, and it becomes more and more difficult for the addict to get any stimulation at all from his addictants.

The onset of this predominantly negative period of withdrawals is usually identified by the patient and all concerned as the "onset of the present illness." This phase of the disease may be preceded, however, by a prolonged period of hyperactivity or other stimulatory symptoms. Even after the withdrawal reactions have become predominant, the individual may still experience periods of elation and stimulation, although less and less frequently.

The negative states, or withdrawal levels of reaction, cover a wide gamut of human ill health. They span both mental and physical diseases, since in actuality these are not distinct, totally separate entities, but rather parts of the same overall spectrum. Because of the many and varied symptoms involved, patients with such withdrawal reactions are frequently tagged "neurotics" by their physicians. Many physicians lack the theoretical framework within which to understand this disease.

In the following chapters, five common problems associated with food and chemical susceptibility are reviewed: headache, arthritis, fatigue, "brain-fag," and depression. Many other common or rare illnesses, however, can be associated with withdrawal reactions. It might be helpful, therefore, before proceeding with specific cases, to review the kinds of withdrawal reactions frequently seen by a clinical ecologist.

Localized Withdrawal Symptoms (Minus-one Reactions)

The first stage of negative reaction, minus-one, includes all of the *localized* withdrawal symptoms. In other words, these are physical problems which only occur in one distinct part or organ of the body.

There are six major kinds of localized reactions:

1. Upper Respiratory Symptoms. These include inflammation of the nasal membranes (rhinitis), sinus problems, conjunctivitis and other eye or ear diseases, and problems associated with these, such as coughing, frequent clearing of the throat, raising of excessive phlegm, postnasal drip, and nasal obstruction. Other eye problems include an abnormal sensitivity to light (photophobia), blurring or dimness of vision, and excessive crying or itchiness around the eyes. Ear problems may include discharge from the ear, earache, deafness (especially of the intermittent kind), and inner or middle ear problems, such as vertigo, dizziness, lightheadedness, giddiness, or floating sensations.

Intense itching of the nose, palate, eyes, and ears, as well as profuse mucus production from the nose, eyes, throat, and sinuses, is often the result of some specific food allergy. Itching of the eyes, on the other hand, more frequently indicates susceptibility to particles in the air, especially pollen. Nasal polyps are often the result of drug sensitivity, especially, it seems, to aspirin.

2. Lower Respiratory Symptoms. The lower respiratory system includes the vocal cords (larynx), the bronchial tubes, and the lungs. Vocal cord symptoms range from hoarseness to periodic voice loss. Coughing and bronchitis often occur and can be either seasonal or year-round, constant or intermittent, mild or severe.

Some respiratory symptoms can be the forerunners of bronchial asthma. One of these is a form of difficult breathing called "sighing dyspnea" in which the patient experiences difficulty or distress in breathing, frequently accompanied by sighing-type noises. This condition often is regarded as the sign of a neurotic or nervous person. However, it also characterizes the patient with chemical or food allergy and can be the prelude to asthma.

The most common causes of hoarseness and loss of voice are reactions to specific foods. Tobacco smoke, however, is a very common cause of persistent coughing in patients who do not have asthma. Even nonsmokers can be affected in this way if subjected to someone else's smoke. Bronchial asthma may also be caused by exposure to inhaled particles, chemicals, animal danders, or drugs.

3. Dermatologic (Skin) Reactions. This category includes such problems as eczema, itching, and hives. Many cases of eczema are caused by environmental exposures and most are characterized by itchiness. Exceptions are some cases of acne, psoriasis, and certain rare skin diseases which may or may not respond to ecologic management.

The most common sites for skin problems caused by food allergy are the neck, ears, and, in general, the folds of the body. Reactions to ointments are a common source of skin problems, which is ironic, since many ointments which are used to treat skin problems actually induce contact-type reactions.

Hives, or wheals, are commonly caused by drugs, and somewhat less frequently by specific foods. This type of reaction to drugs, such as penicillin, is of course common and well known. Less well known are similar reactions to chemical or biological drugs, which can be caused by both the active ingredient in the drug and by dyes, chemical preservatives, or other constituents.

4. *Gastrointestinal Problems.* Such illnesses include problems of the stomach or gut, such as diarrhea, constipation, gas, bloating, abdominal distress, nausea, vomiting, ulcerative colitis, and regional ileitis. In fact, any chronic or intermittent stomach or intestinal problem of unknown origin may have its basis in the environment, particularly in the foods one eats.

Peptic ulcers, which kill almost 6,000 Americans a year, can be either caused or perpetuated by responses to particular foods. There is no universal diet that can be given as a mass prescription for this problem: the proper diet for the individual depends on his particular response to foods. For example, milk, which has often been given as a treatment for ulcers, frequently turns out to be a *cause* of such reactions.

Specific food responses may also mimic gallbladder disease, appendicitis, and even intestinal obstruction. Colitis and ileitis are most often caused by food allergies. It is tragic to remove parts of the digestive system by surgery before food allergy has been ruled out in each and every case.

5. *Genitourinary System Symptoms.* These symptoms include urgency or frequency of urination, proneness to urinary tract infections, and some prostate trouble. The most common cause of such problems is foods. Specific foods can also cause an excessive discharge from the female organs, in cases where infection is not involved. (As a side note, the presence of infection does not rule out the parallel problem of allergy. The two problems can and do occur together, since allergic irritation can prepare the ground for a subsequent infection by microorganisms.)

6. *Cardiovascular System Symptoms.* The cardiovascular system includes the heart and the circulatory system. The principal problems encountered include edema (swelling), arrhythmia (irregular heartbeats), and hypertension. Swelling and water retention, especially when it is generalized through the body, tend to have an allergic basis. Some local swelling can also occur: For example, edema around the eyelids is fairly common, resulting in the characteristic "allergic shiners" and a lacklustre appearance of the eyes.

High blood pressure (hypertension) and cardiac irregularities have long been associated with reactions to specific foods. Less commonly, they are caused by environmental chemicals and drugs. The cardiovascular effects, although localized to one anatomical system, take place through the body. They thus serve as a kind of bridge between localized and systemic reactions, which we shall consider next.

Systemic Withdrawal Symptoms (Minus-two, -three, and -four Reactions)

In the following chapters, five kinds of systemic withdrawal manifestations are described. These are among the most troublesome and mistreated forms of environmental disease. In the following paragraphs, the overall scope of systemic problems related to the withdrawal stage will be surveyed and an overview provided of the complexity of the problem.

HEADACHE (MINUS-TWO REACTION)
The pain may be localized in one part of the head, or it may be generalized. It may occur with or without nausea, vomiting, visual disturbances, or muscle involvement. It can meet the classical picture of migraine, with visions of flashing lights, and a general malaise. It is frequently accompanied by blurring of vision, weakness of the limbs, or pains in the nape, shoulders, and upper back—for this reason headache qualifies as a systemic, not just a local, problem.

Sometimes a headache is followed by a period of relative good health in which no pain is present. This "breathing space" tends to occur in the earlier stages of the problem, however. As it develops, headaches tend to become increasingly common and more severe.

MUSCLE ACHES AND PAINS (MINUS-TWO REACTION)
Both fatigue and headache are commonly associated with myalgia, or muscle pain. The frequency of this association has led some doctors to refer to it as the "tension-fatigue syndrome." While the term suggests that the syndrome is caused by psychological tension, it is most commonly related to food and chemical susceptibility.

Myalgia, although frequently centered in the nape of the neck, may involve many other muscles. Muscle spasms (such as torticollis, lumbago, and sciatica), muscle cramps, aches, pains and weakness, chest pains (through the involvement of muscles of the chest wall), and abdominal pains are all possible symptoms.

Ignorance of the allergic basis of these pains sometimes leads to incorrect diagnoses of pleurisy, appendicitis, and even heart attacks.

JOINT ACHES AND PAINS (MINUS-TWO REACTIONS)
Arthritis of all types, arthralgia (joint aches), joint swelling, and bursitis all frequently have an allergic basis and can be controlled through altering the environment, as the case histories will make clear.

FATIGUE (MINUS-TWO REACTION)

By allergic fatigue is meant tiredness which is unrelieved by the customary, or even an excessive, amount of rest. Fatigue is possibly the most common systemic symptom caused by allergy.* Although there are many variations on this theme, fatigue resulting from food allergy is usually at its worst in the morning and gradually improves as the day advances. This is due to the daily schedule of the food addict. Allergic fatigue is associated with general weakness, drowsiness, and the sensation of heavy limbs. It is also frequently associated with other allergic responses, such as swelling, headache, irritability, and low levels of confusion and depression.

Fatigue caused by exposure to pollen and other inhalants is also known, but is usually seasonal and easier to recognize and control.

BRAIN-FAG OR IMPAIRED THINKING ABILITY (MINUS-THREE REACTIONS)

"Brain-fag" is a designation for a rather severe, but unfortunately common, condition. This is the minus-three category, and its symptoms are *systemic*, but predominantly "mental" rather than physical. Such patients suffer from mild depression, with sadness, moodiness, and sullenness; mental confusion and disturbed thinking; impaired memory and reading comprehension; minimal brain dysfunction; indecisiveness; mental lapses, including aphasia and blackouts; and, in general, the whole gamut of "neuroses," hypochondria, and so-called psychosomatic illnesses.

All of these problems can occur, but more commonly only a few of them are found in a single individual. The condition may get somewhat better for a while, or it may change back to a minus-two reaction (systemic and *physical*). But the general tendency is for it to linger or to get worse with the passage of time.

In a sense this is the most characteristic form of food and chemical allergy, for it represents the "bottom-of-the-barrel" for a great many advanced cases.

SEVERE DEPRESSION, WITH OR WITHOUT ALTERED CONSCIOUSNESS (MINUS-THREE AND MINUS-FOUR REACTIONS)

Depression straddles the fence between minus-three and minus-four reactions. In its most severe form, the patient experiences stupor, lethargy, and impaired responsiveness. Childish thinking, disorientation, amnesia, paranoid feelings, and even hallucinations may occur. Apathy, lethargy, and stupor are seen. The patient at this extreme level may lapse into a coma.

---

* Such fatigue can also have other causes, such as anemia, cancer, or endocrine dysfunctions. These diseases must be ruled out in any study of this problem.

The minus-four stage also includes the various forms of "psychosis," including manic-depressive disease and schizophrenia.

Most allergy patients never reach this extreme level of depression. However, once they do, it is difficult to treat them or even to obtain a history. In the latter stages of this kind of illness, a patient often cannot take care of himself and often cannot even give his correct name, much less a coherent history of his illness. The cause of the problem can usually be detected, but a great deal of family support is necessary for complete recovery. Schizophrenics who have become used to, and comfortable with, state welfare support or institutionalized care often make poor patients and may not be properly motivated to get better.

It should be obvious, then, that the scope of environmental disease is great. It includes many of the common chronic ailments which send people to doctors, although of course other causes of these ailments are also possible and should be investigated along with food and chemical susceptibility. It would be impossible in a book such as this to give a more thorough treatment of all of these syndromes. Instead, four common illnesses will be discussed at greater length below. The first is a physical ailment—headache—which is often erroneously diagnosed as psychosomatic in origin. The second is a physical, systemic illness—rheumatoid arthritis. The third is "brain-fag," the most characteristic form of illness caused by food and chemical allergy. Finally, the most severe form of the problem, depression (which straddles minus-three and minus-four categories), is examined in greater depth.

The case histories in each chapter should add a human aspect to the rather bare bones of theory and show how even the seemingly incurable cases can be properly diagnosed and treated, and how many patients have been enabled to start leading normal lives once more.

12
Headache (Minus-two Reaction)

Headache is commonly the result of food or chemical susceptibility. A large proportion of head pains, including even the worst forms of migraine, are simply due to allergic reactions. There is no need for a person to suffer for years on end with persistent headaches when the cause of these disorders can often be identified and relieved by eliminating certain common substances from the environment.

The idea that specific foods could cause headache is not new. As early as 1905, the Australian medical pioneer, Dr. Francis Hare, reported that head pain could be the result of eating incompatible foods.[1] This observation was not pursued at the time by the medical profession. In 1927, two prominent American allergists, Drs. Albert G. Rowe and Warren T. Vaughan, both published articles implicating specific foods as the cause of allergic headaches.[2,3]

My own first medical paper, published in August, 1935, dealt with the subject of "Allergy in Migraine-like Headaches."[4] In it, Dr. John M. Sheldon and I, both then associated with the University of Michigan Medical School, observed that two-thirds of the migraine patients at the University Hospital in Ann Arbor obtained relief of their headaches by eliminating various foods from their diet.

These results were certainly better than those achieved by conventional medicine. Today, however, even better results can be achieved through the diagnosis of chemical susceptibility and of some common food allergies, which had not then been identified.

Allergic headaches do not discriminate in the site they attack. Every conceivable kind of headache—bilateral, frontal, as well as those radiating into the nape of the neck or the jaws—has been identified and controlled on the basis of clinical ecology.

123

Since certain physicians have promoted alleged "antiheadache diets," it is important to emphasize again that there is no mass-applicable shortcut to controlling such painful syndromes. What affects one patient does not trouble the next. There is simply no substitute for working out one's own food allergy picture, using the methods explained later in this book.

A patient is rarely aware of the environmental source of his illness. He may see no relation between eating and headache, since the effects can be delayed. Or he may know that his headache is somehow related to his food intake, but that intake is so complex and varied that uncovering the actual source may seem like an impossibility. Or he may know that a particular food *relieves* his headache pain, not realizing that it may also cause it and that the "relief" meal is nothing but his maintenance dose.

The physical manner in which allergies cause headache is not entirely known, nor is this information crucial to either patient or physician. One possible explanation is that allergic reactions often cause water retention, or edema. When bellies or ankles become bloated, this is discomforting and disfiguring. But when the brain swells, it pushes against the inflexible skull, and pain results.

This theory receives support from the observations of Dr. Bernard S. Zussman, of Memphis, Tennessee, who had an allergic patient with a hole in his skull from an earlier brain operation. Whenever this patient ate a food to which he was allergic, his brain would literally swell and expand slightly out of the hole. Perhaps patients who speak of feeling "soggy" or "water-logged" in their heads are being more scientifically accurate than they imagine.

CASE STUDY: HEADACHE

Joan Kowan was one of my earliest and most difficult headache patients. She had been a student nurse until she was expelled from the nurses' training program for poor attendance. Her constant, severe headaches had prevented her from being able to keep up with her classmates. So severe were these attacks that, in desperation, she had consented to two brain operations. They were complete failures, and the surgeons could find nothing organically wrong.

In my office, she was found to be highly sensitive to milk. By avoiding milk and dairy products in all of their forms, she was able to control her headache problem and return to school. As time went by, however, it became increasingly difficult for her to avoid all forms of milk. She lived in a college dormitory and ate institutional food. While the regular cook had cooperated with her requests, he was not always there. For example, her vegetables were cooked and set aside before butter was added. A substitute cook, however, did not do this, and Joan unknowingly ate the buttered vegetables. Within an hour, she suddenly fell to the floor in the nurse's station, overcome by violent head pains. The cause of this reaction was traced, in retrospect, to the seemingly insignificant amount of butter on her vegetables. Such inadvertent exposures to milk were fairly common and most troublesome.

To alleviate the pain, she began to take codeine tablets, until she became addicted to them. She also became dependent on other pain-killers to which milk sugar was added as a filler. Thus, while these drugs appeared to give relief, they were actually perpetuating her basic problem.

Miss Kowan was so amazingly susceptible to milk that I thought it would be worth recording some of the features of her case for the medical record. She agreed to take an EEG (electroencephalogram) test, which records brain waves, while drinking a minute amount of milk.

To make the test "blind," she was given two drops of milk in a glass of water. This, at least, is what she was told she was receiving. Actually, the first sample she chose contained several drops of an inert antacid, aluminum hydroxide (Amphojel), in a glass of water. The water became slightly cloudy, just as if it had had milk added. She drank this with fear and trembling, since she anticipated one of her characteristic headaches. Nothing happened. She was then given two drops of actual milk in a glass of water, but she was told she was receiving more of the previous substance. This time she rapidly went into agonizing pain. In her writhing, she pulled herself free of the EEG machine, ruining that part of the experiment.

Her case made clear, however, the ability of even small amounts of an incriminated substance to cause severe and chronic headaches.

Miss Kowan eventually managed to get her allergy under control and to graduate. Years later I received a letter from her. She had obtained an excellent position with a large manufacturing concern and had a good work record, with few absences. "Since you saw me last," she wrote, "I have not faltered in my quest for a new future."

CASE STUDY: HEADACHE AND DRUG ADDICTION

Edward Rideout had had headaches for many years. In his childhood, these were fairly infrequent. In his youth, the attacks were accompanied by other symptoms, such as nausea and vomiting. After an hour or two of sleep, he would feel better. Like Joan Kowan, Rideout constantly resorted to pain-killers and became addicted to these drugs. Eventually, he became addicted to a morphine-derived medication.

Each of Rideout's headaches followed a characteristic pattern. His headache would come on suddenly, he would become nauseated, and would begin to vomit. This attack would be accompanied by nervousness, restlessness, hyperactivity, and sensitivity to light.

Midway through one of these terrible attacks, he would rush to the nearest emergency room for an injection of his morphine medication. Eventually, in desperation, he, too, consented to a brain operation designed to ease the pain. Again, this accomplished nothing.

Treatment with comprehensive environmental control brought dramatic changes in his condition. During the withdrawal period of the water fast, he had to be given some morphine medication to relieve the unbearable pain. By the third or fourth day of the fast, however, the pain subsided, and the medication was discontinued. On the fifth day of withdrawal, Rideout became violently angry at the world. That evening he felt as if he were about to get a headache, but it never came. On the morning of his sixth day of fasting, he woke without a sign of a headache. There was only a slight tenderness in his mid-forehead. During the next ten days, Rideout tested a variety of foods and waters according to the procedures of the Ecology Unit. The results of these tests finally exposed the root causes of this man's lifelong headache problem.

He turned out to be susceptible to the following substances:

One form of tap water: bad headache
Cantaloupe: slight headache, which lasted half an hour
Corn and corn sugar: headache on first test; "thick feeling across forehead"
     on second test, with some depression
Banana: bad headache
Fish (catfish): severe headache, lasting two days
Rabbit: intense pressure across forehead

Other foods gave no reaction, nor did chemically contaminated meals or other forms of common chemicals. A suitable diet, containing only those items which were tolerated, was devised for him. Leaving the hospital, Rideout was headache-free for the first time in decades. He has continued to make progress, following his diet and adding new items to it whenever possible.

Headaches do not always occur alone, but often accompany other symptoms. These can either be localized symptoms (minus-one), other minus-two reactions, or even more severe minus-three symptoms. Sandra Casey was one of these polysymptomatic patients.

CASE STUDY: HEADACHE AND DEPRESSION

Sandra Casey was twenty-one years old when she entered the Ecology Unit. Her headaches centered around her eyes and forehead. They were steady in nature and accompanied by sensitivity to light. She had these headaches three or four times a month, and each lasted for three or four days. While having a headache, she was unable to sleep or rest yet could take no medication, for medicine seemed to make her depressed.

Miss Casey had been diagnosed as having hypoglycemia (low blood sugar) several months before she came to the unit. She had been on a hypoglycemia diet which consisted of six small, high-protein meals a day. At first she felt much better on this diet, but eventually she became depressed and suicidal. (Doctors see many such cases of alleged hypoglycemia. The symptoms, including marked swings in blood-sugar levels after consumption of corn sugar, may frequently be the result of food allergies, not of true hypoglycemia, a point first noted by Dr. William A. Philpott of Oklahoma City.)

Another problem which Mrs. Casey had was what she called "attacks." The first attack came after she took some hashish at the age of fifteen. She became very cold, and her limbs felt as if they were frozen all day. She thought she were going to die or go insane, yet a physician who examined her declared that there were no permanent effects from the drug.

Since that time, however, she had had frequent sensations of numbness, which would start in her back and radiate over her head. This feeling was quite difficult for her to explain; she said it was similar to having a bucket of cold water poured over one's head. After the attack she became disoriented, depressed, and suicidal.

As stated, this patient's symptoms ranged from localized physical reactions (minus-one) to more profound systemic changes. She complained of sore throat, phlegm in the back of her throat, chest pain, lightheadedness, and dizziness. Her abdominal bloating became so troublesome that she looked as if she were pregnant.

Because of her depression and suicidal tendencies, Sandra had been under the care of a psychiatrist and had been institutionalized for nineteen days. Antidepressive drugs made her even more suicidal. In fact, her suicidal thoughts were becoming obsessive, especially since her husband was a gun collector who kept arms within easy reach around the house.

She reported a craving for sugar and sweet foods in general and said she loved to go through a box of cookies at a single sitting. Not surprisingly, her strongest reactions in testing were to wheat, corn, peas, blueberries, beets and beet sugar, and other commonly eaten foods, taken singly according to the methods of the Ecology Unit. Commercial foods gave her a headache, cumulatively, after five meals.

She left the hospital headache-free and in a normal frame of mind. Her problem was diagnosed as multiple food and chemical susceptibility, and her chances of recovery were excellent, provided she followed the recommended procedures.

Suffice it to say, in summary, that headaches demonstrated to be on an allergic basis may be of any descriptive type—that is, any location, any degree of severity, with or without usual symptoms, nausea, vomiting, or other features. Although allergic headaches are far more commonly demonstrated to be on the basis of reactions to given foods and/or environmental chemical exposures, they may also be related to such allergens as house dust, pollens, and sometimes drugs. Indeed, I have seen patients whose treatment with such pain-relieving drugs as codeine accentuates their headaches.

As mentioned earlier, allergic headaches were described over a half century ago. Under these circumstances, there is no excuse for patients to be told to "live" with their headaches. When headache patients are investigated by means of proper techniques to demonstrate their environmental causes, to which susceptibility exists, most cases may be readily diagnosed and treated in the absence of drug therapy.

Finally, although headaches are sometimes said to be on a psychogenic basis, I have not been able to demonstrate such a relationship. If this exists, it must be exceedingly rare.

13

Arthritis and Related Muscle and Joint Pains (Minus-two Reactions)

Arthritis is one of the most common systemic physical diseases in advanced countries. There are two main types, rheumatoid and osteoarthritis; rheumatoid arthritis may begin at any age, but usually is found earlier in a person's life than osteoarthritis or degenerative arthritis, which is more characteristic of older people.

So-called traumatic arthritis may develop into either rheumatoid or osteoarthritis. And mixed arthritis, with features of both rheumatoid and osteoarthritis, is also common. Although any joint or joints may be involved in rheumatoid or osteoarthritis, the joints of the hands are particularly vulnerable. While the terminal finger joints are characteristically affected in osteoarthritis, involvement of the second finger joints and, to a less extent, the knuckles and wrists are characteristically affected in rheumatoid arthritis.

This chapter is principally concerned with rheumatoid arthritis and to a lesser extent with the muscle involvement (allergic myalgia) which so frequently accompanies it. Victims of rheumatoid arthritis, either with or without myalgia (muscle aching), do not need to be reminded that orthodox medicine tends to be at a loss to explain the origin of their illness or to offer effective measures in its treatment, beyond the use of aspirin or other pain-killers. Any considerations of "causes" is usually subject to debate concerning alleged bodily mechanisms. Unfortunately, the causative roles of environmental factors in rheumatoid arthritis or myalgia are usually not considered seriously.

By contrast, clinical ecology, from the beginning of its involvement with muscle and joint aches and pains, has attempted to understand and pinpoint responsible environmental factors. As with other environmentally related illnesses described in this book, the role played by environmental exposures in instances of rheumatoid arthritis is highly individualized in nature, based on a given person's susceptibility to such a food. For instance, given foods are not incriminated as environmental causes of arthritis in all rheumatoids, nor is there any universal treatment likely to benefit all cases. Indeed, from the standpoint of the application of clinical ecology to this illness and related conditions, there is no substitute for the patient's unravelling of a highly individualized ecologic problem by means of the methods described in this book.

Although there had been earlier references to the relationship of foods to arthritis, the first definitive and convincing presentation of this subject occurred in 1949, when Michael Zeller published an article: "Rheumatoid Arthritis—Food Allergy as a Factor," in the *Annals of Allergy*. Zeller was the first to demonstrate a cause-and-effect relationship between the intake of specific foods and the onset of acute symptoms of arthritis.[1] Zeller carefully pointed out that not all patients with rheumatoid arthritis responded to the approach based on the exclusion of incriminated foods. I had worked closely with Dr. Zeller, observing several of his cases at first hand, and confirmed his clinical observations in my own practice. We discussed foods as major factors in arthritis and myalgia in the book we wrote jointly with Rinkel, *Food Allergy* (1951).[2]

Although approximately 1,000 cases of rheumatoid arthritis have been studied by me from the standpoint of food allergy during the last three decades, there was nothing to report in addition to Zeller's observations until recent years. But as I became increasingly aware of the chemical susceptibility problem, most of the patients who had failed to respond satisfactorily to food allergy management turned out to have at least a part of their arthritis on the basis of susceptibility to environmental chemicals. Consequently, the ecologic management of rheumatoid arthritis due to both foods and environmental chemicals was updated in 1976.[3] The approaches and techniques of clinical ecology offer scientifically founded hope to the great majority of rheumatoid arthritics.

When Dr. Kendall Gerdes, now of Denver, Colorado, was associated with me in training in clinical ecology, we sent follow-up questionnaires to over 200 cases of hospitalized arthritics, who had been managed ecologically. Both the cases of rheumatoid arthritis and osteoarthritis did equally well as a result of avoiding incriminated environmental exposures. It might also be added that other types of arthritis are also environmentally related. Other rheumatoid states, such as Reiter's syndrome, ankylosing spondylitis, and psoriatric arthritis, have also been studied ecologically, but in insufficient numbers from which to draw conclusions. My Ecology Unit is currently involved in a prospective study of rheumatoid arthritis of the hands in which measurements of the size, tenderness, and mobility of affected joints are taken prior to and following fasting and challenges with specific foods and environmental chemicals. The results of this study should be available in the near future.

CASE STUDY: RHEUMATOID ARTHRITIS WITH DEPRESSION

Helen Jones, a 35-year-old nurse, had suffered from sinus problems since childhood. She had also had periodic episodes of gas, bloating, indigestion, and, occasionally, diarrhea. Within the previous five years, Mrs. Jones had experienced increasing fatigue and the need for excessive amounts of sleep. Seven months after moving into a new house, she developed tendonitis of the wrists, soon followed by arthritis of the right shoulder and knee. After giving birth, she developed arthritis of the hands, feet, knees, and shoulders, as well as progressive weakness and muscular cramps in the right calf.

These painful joint and muscle syndromes were accompanied by other withdrawal-type illnesses such as fatigue, irritability, and depression.

In desperation, Mrs. Jones submitted to an operation on her right knee to relieve the pain and crippling inflammation. This procedure brought some temporary relief, but soon her left knee was in just as bad condition as the other had been. By the time she was admitted to the hospital for comprehensive environmental control, her left knee and wrist were swollen, tender, and inflamed, with sharply limited and painful motion. The knee which had been operated upon was still swollen, but no longer inflamed.

When Mrs. Jones fasted and avoided smoking and other suspected environmental factors, such as air pollution and household chemicals, she developed a severe withdrawal-type headache, but her arthritis improved. By the end of five days of fasting, she was able to walk without crutches for the first time in months.

When single foods, known not to have been significantly contaminated with chemical additives, were returned to her diet, reactions occurred to the following:

Corn: 10 minutes, severe arthritic pain

Cane: 15 minutes, pains in knees and hands plus abdominal cramps

Apple: 30 minutes, abdominal distress and arthritic pain

Lamb: 35 minutes, severe arthritic pain

Orange: 40 minutes, intermittent waves of apprehension and depression followed by progressively severe arthritic pain

Grape: 40 minutes, increased dizziness and arthritic pain

Egg: 45 minutes, gradual onset of arthritic pain

Wheat: 1 hour, stiffness of knee; accentuated immediately after second feeding 1 hour later

Pork: 1 hour, gradual onset of fatigue and depression with residual increased arthritic pain

Rice: 1 hour, slowly increasing joint stiffness, fatigue, and irritability
Lobster tail: 3 hours, lightheadedness with increased stiffness of joints
Beef: 3½ hours, gradual onset of arthritic swelling and pain

All other commonly eaten foods were tolerated with no flare-ups of her symptoms, but when tomato juice, which had been tolerated in its uncontaminated form, was given to her from a phenol-lined can, she reacted with stiffness of the joints after fifteen minutes, followed by rapidly increasing fatigue, irritability, and depression.

Upon returning home, Mrs. Jones was instructed to use only nonchlorinated water for drinking and cooking, to avoid all incriminated foods, and to rotate the use of chemically less contaminated foods.

She continued to improve steadily at home on this program but experienced mild recurrences of symptoms from massive exposure to plastics. During the past several years, there have been no troublesome arthritic symptoms. At the present time, she is able to eat pork, beef, lobster tail, wheat, egg, cane, and lamb once a week. Accidental breaks in the avoidance of corn sugar (dextrose) have been followed by bouts of irritability and depression but not arthritis. Corn as a cereal has not been tried. Mrs. Jones still finds that it is necessary to eat chemically less contaminated (organic) food to remain free of arthritis pains.

Several features stand out from this case. One can see that over a period of years, Mrs. Jones' ecologic problems were progressing from minus-one symptoms (sinus problems, indigestion) to minus-two, especially arthritis and fatigue. At the same time, she was already entering a minus-three phase with the development of depression as a result of food susceptibility.

It is also noteworthy how quickly Mrs. Jones reacted to her test foods. For example, she came down with severe arthritic pains only ten minutes after eating corn and fifteen minutes after eating cane sugar. Generally speaking, the more severe a person's arthritis, the more rapidly he will react to an incriminated food or chemical exposure.

CASE STUDY: ARTHRITIS WITH MYALGIA

Patricia Engel was a skilled pianist and violinist, thirty years of age, who had been well until moving into an all gas-equipped house. At the same time she had changed most of her wardrobe from natural to synthetic fabrics. Within a four-to-five-month period she noticed that she needed rest periods during the day. She also suffered from increasing levels of morning fatigue. Soon this was followed by unexplained muscle soreness.

Miss Engel took a trip to Europe. After being exposed to excessive amounts of motor exhaust while traveling, however, she developed chills and arthritic pains of the neck and shoulders. Another similar episode occurred after she disembarked in New York City when she ran into heavy traffic fumes. But two weeks after returning to her apartment, with its gas-fired range and water heater, generalized joint and muscle aching and pain incapacitated her. The pain started in her shoulders and spine and then spread rapidly to her fingers, hips, knees, ankles, and other joints.

Conventionally minded doctors treated her with aspirin and another nonaspirin pain-killer. Soon she was given cortisone therapy. After three years of this, however, she developed a cataract, whereupon the drug was discontinued. She also received indomethacin (Indocin) and gold therapy, an experimental form of arthritis treatment. Nothing stopped the spread of the disease. By this point, she was so crippled that she had to abandon her career as a musician, since she could no longer play the piano or violin.

Upon admission to the hospital under my care, she fasted and suffered headaches and muscle and joint pains as withdrawal symptoms. These symptoms soon cleared, and her joint movement increased. Miss Engel was then tested with chemically less contaminated health foods. Her reactions, listed in the order of their rapidity of onset, were as follows:

Corn: 30 minutes, sleepiness; 1 hour, restlessness; 3 hours, fatigue and sensitive joints, with generalized myalgia and arthralgia the following morning

Tomato: 30 minutes, knees, hands, and wrists more tight

Peas: 30 minutes, arms, shoulders, and fingers tightened and more sensitive

Beets and beet sugar: 1 hour, restless legs and increasing generalized stiffness

Lamb: 2 hours, hoarseness, followed by chilling and progressive fatigue and arthritic pains

Rice: 2 hours, tightness and stiffness of knees and wrists

Wheat: 4 hours, restless legs with residual muscle and joint stiffness

Milk: 4 hours, stiffness of joints with residual generalized joint stiffness and soreness

Beef: 8 hours, aching joints with residual pain in joints

When Miss Engel was fed regular supermarket foods, which had been tolerated in their organic form, after the third such meal she awoke during the night with extreme stiffness and chills, all her joints being so sore that she had to be helped out of bed.

Upon returning home, she avoided all of her incriminated foods, and chlorinated water, and by following the Rotary Diversified Diet (Chap. 18), she remained well. Within a week, however, her arthritis gradually returned. This was tremendously disappointing, especially since she had previously removed her gas stove. She did notice, however, that she felt better when she was outside the house and became increasingly worse the more time she spent inside.

She therefore had her gas-fired heating system removed and replaced it with electric heaters and also had the gas pipes removed from the walls. She made her bedroom into a pollution-free "oasis" (Chap. 20) and then reintroduced questionable items one at a time. She was found to be susceptible to polyester bedsheets, living-room curtains, and several other plastic and synthetic materials. The finish on the doors of her kitchen cabinets was suspected, and there was definite improvement when it was removed.

At the present time, Miss Engel is free of muscle and joint pain, but there remains some impaired motion in the left wrist, due to the destruction of tissue caused when her illness was uncontrolled. She also gets a mild increase in arthritic symptoms before her monthly period, after housekeeping, when the pine trees in her yard are putting out new growth, and when she is working in the yard. However, there is simply no comparison between the minor problems which she has now and the crippled patient whom we admitted to the hospital a few years ago.

Patricia Engel is just the sort of patient whose case could not have been fully understood in the 1940s or early 1950s, because much of her illness was caused by chemical susceptibility. Even such a seemingly innocuous material as the varnish on her kitchen cabinets was contributing to her arthritis and had to be modified or removed before she could get significantly better.

Few diseases are as pathetic as rheumatoid arthritis in children. This problem often starts innocently enough as a swelling in a knuckle or finger, spreads to other parts of the body, and finally leaves the child a cripple for life. It is often accompanied by swollen lymph nodes (glands), enlarged spleen, fever, profuse sweating, and anemia. Conventional medicine recognizes no agreed-upon cause or effective treatment for this ailment.

CASE HISTORY: JUVENILE ARTHRITIS

Kelly Johnson was a nine-year-old schoolgirl when she developed arthritis of the right ankle in the spring of 1970. This was followed by migration of the arthritis to both knees and ankles. Aspirin was the only treatment given until an operation (called a synovectomy) was performed on the right knee, in order to allow it to move more freely.

Four months later, the partially crippled child was hospitalized for food and chemical testing. Examination revealed swelling and limitation of motion in both knees, as well as a scar from the previous operation. Upon beginning the period of fasting, Kelly experienced nausea and headache as withdrawal effects. Progressive improvement occurred, however, so that after four days of fasting her joints were more mobile and less painful than they had been in many months.

Severe recurrences of arthritic pain, swelling, and other symptoms was associated with the ingestion of the following chemically less contaminated (organic) foods:

Rice: 2 hours, stomachache; 9 hours, itching
Chicken: 2½ hours, pains in elbows and hands
Pork: 3 hours, stomachache; 14 hours, joint stiffness
Beef: 3 hours, chest pain and residual stiffness
Potato: 3 hours, right-shoulder pain
Wheat: 3½ hours, itching
Corn: 5 hours, itching; 10 hours, swollen extremities
Milk: 9½ hours, mild itching of skin only
Beet: 14 hours, swollen, stiff hands and feet

In contrast to some of the earlier cases, Kelly's symptoms generally came on hours after the food ingestion test. Since another meal may have intervened between the ingestion of corn, milk, or beet and the development of symptoms, it was often necessary to repeat tests in order to make sure that a given food resulted in a given symptom. This is the kind of test which is extremely difficult to do outside a specialized hospital setting.

Other commonly eaten foods were all test-negative. Kelly went home in good condition and remained well on the diet we devised for her until the gas-fired furnace was turned on that fall. This was followed by a flare-up in her arthritis. She was therefore moved to an all-electric house. Since then, Kelly has remained symptom-free, adhering well to her dietary program. Other than some physiotherapy for pain in the operated knee, she needs no therapy—not even aspirin—at the present time.

CASE STUDY: JUVENILE ARTHRITIS

Another case of juvenile arthritis, this time in an even younger child, was that of Louise Holmes. Louise was only three-and-a-half when she came to the Ecology Unit. At the age of two, she had begun to complain of joint pain and had started to run an incessant fever. She had a rash. Studies by a local hospital led to a diagnosis of juvenile rheumatoid arthritis. Aspirin was prescribed and for over a year Louise was brought for weekly visits to the hospital to have her salicylate (aspirin) levels measured. She also was taken regularly to a famous Midwest clinic, but no demonstrable cause or effective treatment had been found for her condition. She had to be carried into the Ecology Unit.

On beginning the program, she was taken off her aspirinlike medicine.

During the fast, Louise experienced a day of vomiting (withdrawal reactions), but after three days of fasting her joint pains completely subsided, and she began walking normally—something she had not done in over a year.

During the next eleven days, Louise was given twenty-six foods to test in their relatively uncontaminated forms. She had strong flare-ups of symptoms after eating carrots, eggs, and chicken, and somewhat less severe reactions to pork, cherry, corn, orange, grape, beef, apple, rice, cane, milk, cod, potato, and honey.

For example, eggs (one of her favorite foods) was followed, about two hours later, with the following reactions: the child said her legs were hurting, and when she was asked where, she pointed to her feet. When eating carrots, she at first reported that she loved them and was in a very happy mood. After 40 minutes, however, she asked for a pillow to sit on because her seat hurt. She soon had a "tummy ache" and loose bowel movement. After one hour, she reported that her knees hurt and pointed specifically to her left knee. She asked her mother, plaintively, "Why does my knee hurt?" Soon she was crying bitterly about the pain in both her knees and was holding her throat. (She had had a polyp removed from her throat the year before.)

Other foods gave no such reactions, however, and the child quickly recovered from these temporary food responses. Kelly left the hospital on her own two feet, completely off her previous medication, and with no pain. There was virtually no swelling in her joints. Since then she has occasionally had intermittent mild swelling in her knee, but without any pain. Her parents have done a good job of keeping incriminated foods out of her diet and of discovering other potential sources of reactions in the environment.

At the other extreme of the spectrum, the clinical ecology approach can also benefit those arthritic patients who are on in years or whose problems are longstanding.

CASE STUDY: ARTHRITIS WITH RHINITIS

Charles Lakerman was a 78-year-old retired businessman who had had rhinitis for the past thirty years and mild intermittent arthritis of the hands for almost a decade. In the fall of 1967, he had developed acute arthritis of the hands, followed by involvement of the right elbow, shoulders, knees, and right hip. Aspirin was the only medication he had received.

At the time of his hospitalization for environmental testing, his hands were red, swollen, and inflamed, with very little motion in the joints. He was barely able to eat and refused to shake hands.

Under the program of comprehensive environmental control, Lakerman's arthritis became progressively better, without his suffering any withdrawal effects. All of his joints were comfortable at the end of five days of fasting, although some residual swelling of the hands persisted.

Individual food ingestion tests resulted in the following reactions:

Corn: 3 hours, nausea and abdominal distress followed by spontaneous diarrhea; 6 hours, recurrence of arthritic pains of hands and left shoulder

Wheat: 3½ hours, watery eyes and running nose; 12 hours, painful right knee upon awakening

Beets and beet sugar: 13 hours, slight aching of ankle upon awakening: a new joint involvement

All other commonly eaten foods were test-negative, nor did he react to the commercial forms of such foods.

Mr Lakerman remained symptom-free at the time of his hospital discharge and experienced no evidence of reaction upon returning home to follow his new diet. After eight months of freedom from arthritis, he tolerated wheat when it was returned to his diet once in five days for several months. However, he experienced a gradual recurrence of mild arthritis of the knees and hands as he increased his intake of wheat to twice daily, corn to three times per week, and began the regular use of beet sugar. All symptoms subsided when he returned to his former diet restrictions, and he has remained free of arthritic pains ever since then.

Many cases of rheumatoid arthritis also have a coexisting muscle involvement referred to as allergic myalgia. This may start either before or following the onset of joint involvement. Allergic myalgia may be acute or chronic, localized or generalized. It tends to be characterized by painful, tender muscles and sometimes presents as cramps or muscle spasms. I first described this condition in 1951.[4] Myalgia of ecologic origin also occurs frequently in the absence of arthritis, in association with headache and fatigue. The postural muscles of the nape, back, chest, and legs are most commonly involved.

Although the causative roles of foods in individually studied cases of rheumatoid arthritis and myalgia have been documented for thirty years, there has been practically no recognition of these findings as taught by rheumatologists in most medical centers. The record shows clearly that of 1,000 cases of rheumatoid arthritis studied during the past three decades, specific foods have been demonstrated in most of them and environmental chemicals in many of them.

14

Fatigue (Minus-two Reaction) and Brain-fag (Minus-three Reaction)

The term *brain-fag* is unfamiliar to most readers. Brain-fag refers to a particular aspect of the environmental disease problem and in fact characterizes the very serious minus-three level. Brain-fag is marked by confused thinking, moodiness, unexplained sadness, and apathy. Frequently, the individual with this phase of the problem cannot concentrate and may find it difficult to express himself. The term itself was first used in this context by an astute patient, and I have adopted it to refer to what may be the most characteristic part of food and chemical susceptibility.

We all know, of course, what fatigue is. Normal people experience it when they have exerted a great deal of energy. Others, however, experience fatigue on an allergic basis. In other words, their tiredness is not related to any particular exertion on their part, is unrelieved by rest or sleep, and is frequently worse in the morning.

Fatigue may also be caused by other disease states, such as chronic infection, metabolic disorders, heart ailments, anemia, dietary deficiencies, or even cancer. If none of these conditions exist, food or chemical allergy should definitely be suspected.

Physical fatigue is a minus-two symptom. It can occur at any age, but not uncommonly afflicts a younger patient than does brain-fag. It can be ruinous for any person who must perform difficult or complicated jobs.

CASE STUDY: PHYSICAL FATIGUE

Rudolph Garvin was a college student, the son of a physician, who wanted to follow in his father's footsteps. His prospects were dim because of his failing grades.

For many years he had suffered from minus-one symptoms, such as rhinitis. He had repeatedly been examined for sinus infections, but none could be found. He also suffered from repeated "colds."

When he entered college, his localized minus-one symptoms gave way to systemic minus-two symptoms: headaches and bouts of extreme tiredness. These would generally come on around 3 P.M. Tiredness and head pain interfered with his ability to study, concentrate, or perform his tasks. He had to try to sneak in some studying before the head-pain problems became too distracting.

Inexplicably, his fatigue fluctuated and was much worse on certain days. In general, his tiredness was associated with bouts of nervousness, tension, and feelings of frustration. He also experienced brain-fag, characterized by impaired reading comprehension and unretentive memory. For instance, he would read his assignment the night before a class but would be unable to remember what he had read the next day. When he first came for ecologic management, his afternoon fatigue had spread to the morning as well. Even after sleeping for eight or nine hours, he awakened tired. Like many such patients, his sleep was restless.

In office tests, two glasses of milk brought on a headache and a feeling of extreme fatigue. He had to lie down until he was able to return home. This was accompanied by stomach upset.

After eating eggs, on another occasion, he suffered a headache after forty minutes. Milk and eggs were daily foods in his diet. He was therefore taken off these items, as well as beef and peanuts, which were both suspected on the basis of his history. After two weeks on the diet, he reported feeling much less tired. He was then instructed to return beef to his diet for three days, followed by peanuts. His headache and fatigue did not reappear. The return of dairy products and eggs, however, was accompanied by a return of his physical fatigue and pain. By eliminating these foods from his diet in all their forms, he recovered his health. After a while, he was able to reintroduce these foods into his diet according to the principles of the Rotary Diversified Diet (Chap. 18). His grades improved, and he was admitted to medical school. Today he is a successful physician.

CASE STUDY: PHYSICAL FATIGUE WITH HEADACHE AND TACHYCARDIA

An even more advanced case was presented by Frederick Eccleson, a student. Eccleson was on the Dean's List—the negative Dean's List for failing students. Although bright, he was flunking out of the scientific institution he had entered with such great expectations a year before.

In high school, Eccleson's heart would suddenly beat at an incredible speed—120 to 160 beats per minute. He was afraid he was about to suffer a heart attack whenever these speedups occurred. In the mornings, he was tired, weak, and irritable. He had perennial headaches, throbbing pains which increased if he even tried to shift position or move his head. Because of this, Eccleson missed about a third of his courses when he entered college. The dean and the school physician considered him a hypochondriac, since no "physical" problem had been discovered.

Eccleson himself was aware of some susceptibilities to foods, including pancakes, eggs, beef, and chocolate. He avoided these items whenever he could, although he had little conception of the degree to which such common foods as beef or eggs penetrate our food supply. He also believed himself to be susceptible to cheese, steak, steak sauce, apple juice, grapefruit, sorghum, and all foods containing baking soda. Eating such foods usually brought on a reaction.

When he was tested in the office with scientific procedures, it was found that he was highly allergic to pork, milk, eggs, potato, beets and beet sugar, and peanuts. Eggs, for instance, brought on severe coughing, shortness of breath, and even vomiting.

By avoiding these incriminated foods entirely, he underwent a transformation. His fatigue and headache went away quickly. One day he popped in to visit me and proudly handed me an official school certificate citing him for "having completed the work of the past quarter with *high honors.*" He had obtained straight A's in all his courses, including those in Analog Computers, Feedback Systems, and Lasers. At the bottom of the photocopy he had handed me he had written simply, "Thank you, Dr. Randolph."

Brain-fag is difficult to describe to those who have not seen it close up. It is a form of *mental* fatigue, a much more serious and debilitating symptom than physical tiredness. Brain-fag is characterized by mental confusion, slowness of thought, lack of initiative and ambition, irritability, occasional loss of sex drive, despondency, as well as bodily fatigue, weakness, and aching.

Some brain-fag patients report a feeling of being slowly poisoned. This becomes grist for some psychiatrists' mill—the fear of poisoning is interpreted as typical "paranoid" thinking. Unconsciously, however, such patients are expressing a truth: chemicals in the environment *are* slowly poisoning them, as are their reactions to commonly eaten foods.

People with brain-fag are more obviously ill than those at the minus-two level. Often called "phobic," they are too dizzy to walk, cannot get out of bed, cannot express their thoughts or remember what they are told. They seem to have lost their desire for life, and sometimes even call themselves the "living dead."

Such patients are almost never properly diagnosed. They have "graduated" to this condition through a number of previous levels of physical and mental distress. They therefore usually have thick medical files, filled with long lists of complaints, many of them seemingly mental in origin. In truth, their medical problems are basically physical in origin (responses to foods or chemicals), but no one realizes this. To their doctors, their family members, and sometimes even themselves, they are classic "hypochondriacs" and attention-seekers.

Such patients are among the prime recipients of mood-altering drugs, electroshock therapy, psychotherapy, and prolonged sermons from assorted well-wishers. None of this does much good, and as time goes by they tend to get progressively sicker. They may eventually graduate to the deep despondency of minus-four: depression, or "psychosis." Others linger at the minus-three level for years, sometimes experiencing temporary remissions. The general course of an untreated ecologic illness, however, is downward.

Since minus-three reactors often graduate from the minus-two category, which includes physical fatigue, the distinction between brain-fag and plain tiredness was difficult to make. The first clear description of both phenomena was made in 1930 by Dr. Albert Rowe, the father of the study of food allergy, who called food-caused fatigue "allergic toxemia." In an article which he wrote on the subject, he gave a good description of some of the mental symptoms which commonly are associated with physical tiredness.

Rowe observed that mental symptoms often alternate with physical symptoms. He quoted a sixteenth-century physician who noted, apropos of asthma, that "there appears a great dulness [sic] and fulness [sic] in the head with a slight headache and great sleepiness before the fit [i.e., asthma attack]."[1] This certainly seems to be an old description of the "modern" disease.

In the 1940s, I was able to confirm many of Rowe's observations and put them in the context of environmental illness. In particular, I differentiated between physical (minus-two) fatigue and mental (minus-three) fatigue, or brain-fag. Why hadn't other doctors seen the same thing? They had, of course, but had misinterpreted the phenomena because of their traditional separation of mental and physical problems. "The majority of allergic individuals with the fatigue syndrome," I wrote in the 1940s, "have been previously diagnosed as 'neurotics.' "[2]

CASE STUDY: BRAIN-FAG AND SEXUAL IMPOTENCE

My original brain-fag case was that of Mr. Carrington. Carrington held a position of responsibility within the United States government. His job entailed a great deal of detail work and a profound knowledge of several unusual fields. His colleagues had looked upon Carrington as a kind of human computer in the days before computers had in fact taken over such arduous tasks.

Over a period of years, Carrington noticed that his capacity for work was diminishing. He kept a special file on his desk of difficult material. He found that he could only work on this material at the most once a week, when his brain was "in full gear." During the rest of the time he suffered from what he himself dubbed "brain-fag"—a term he had come across in his wide reading. I was startled by his use of the term *brain-fag* to describe his illness. When I first heard this word, I thought it was pure slang, but on looking it up in dictionaries, I found that it has been in the English language for a century. I have continued to use it, because it is one of the few descriptive terms which has not been "redefined" in psychiatric dictionaries.

Associated with his brain-fag was sexual impotence and malaise. He had more or less lost his sexual drive. The only way he and his wife could have intercourse was if he took two stiff bourbons on a carefully timed schedule. The bourbon would restore his libido for a short while.

Carrington was in the Library of Congress one day, searching for a clue to his "brain-fag," when he came across the book *Food Allergy*, which I had co-authored with Drs. Rinkel and Zeller in 1951 and in which I had described allergic fatigue. He went straight to a phone book, called me up, and within thirty-six hours had been admitted to the hospital under my care.

Carrington turned out to be violently susceptible to corn. This did not surprise me, since he was from the South and many of his fellow Southerners are similarly susceptible. This helped explain why he was stimulated by bourbon, in which corn is a principal ingredient. When Carrington avoided corn in all its forms, as well as a few other foods to which he was found to be susceptible, he underwent a transformation. Both his work output and his sexual ability improved immediately, and he was soon leading a normal and productive life.

Brain-fag may go untreated or unrecognized in those who lead a sedentary, noncompetitive life. For those in positions of responsibility, where they must compete with other relatively well individuals, brain-fag can be a disaster. Two cases will illustrate the course of treated and untreated ecologic illness.

CASE STUDY: BRAIN-FAG WITH HEADACHE AND RHINITIS

Joseph Robinson was a businessman in his forties, whose position in his company was threatened by increasing ill health. He traced the onset of his sickness to a tonsillectomy. Soon after this operation, persistent nasal stuffiness and a post-nasal drip developed, which did not respond to any medication.

A busy person, Robinson paid little attention to these symptoms. A few years later, he began to get headaches in the front of his forehead. These usually came on an hour or two after the evening meal and persisted for the evening. They were often accompanied by bouts of fatigue, "laziness," and mental exhaustion, which kept him pinned to the living-room couch, unable to move.

At first these problems were restricted to the evening hours and were easily attributed to the difficulty and tension of Robinson's job. Soon, however, the fatigue and mental exhaustion began to creep into his daytime hours as well. He would start to go home early, or rest his head on the desk when he was supposed to be working. His job was in jeopardy when he was first examined for ecologic illness.

A variety of the foods which he ate most commonly, including wheat, milk, eggs, coffee, citrus fruit, legumes, chocolates, various meats, and nuts were eliminated for a week or so. To his amazement, he felt much better, experiencing far less fatigue and no headaches. One by one, these foods were returned to his diet. All of them were tolerated with no return of symptoms except for beef and milk (which are closely related). On the third day of eating beef products, he developed a severe headache which lasted ten hours. He developed a headache half an hour after eating his fourth milk-containing meal. Chocolate also made him feel tired.

With the complete avoidance of beef, milk, and chocolate, all of his symptoms of fatigue, headache, and brain-fag disappeared. As a final test, one month later, he treated himself to a glass of milk. A sharp headache rapidly developed. After about six months, however, he regained tolerance for milk, beef, and their by-products. He was then able to reintroduce them into his diet, provided that he did not have any of them more often than once every four days. He had successfully solved the problem that was ruining his career. In fact, his position in the company improved, and he gained a promotion.

CASE STUDY: BRAIN-FAG WITH MEMORY LOSS AND IRRITABILITY

One characteristic of the brain-fag problem is an acute loss of memory. Norma Tolliver came to me for this problem. A year earlier, she had been pursuing a promising career as a buyer for a large manufacturing concern. Her forte was her outstanding memory. She knew the sizes, colors, weights, and other specifications of the company's products, as well as the names and phone numbers of the shipping lines, manufacturers, and other colleagues by heart. Her employers called her the "walking encyclopedia" and relied upon her to have information at the tips of her fingers.

She never failed to supply the information they sought. Then, without warning, her memory began to fade. A succession of doctors analyzed her problem as psychological in origin and offered a number of imaginative explanations. Tolliver tried desperately to hold onto her position, surrounding herself with thick notebooks filled with data of all sorts. This was a transparent device, and her employers became disillusioned, suspecting her of having tricked them all along. Eventually, she was fired.

Testing in a hospital setting revealed serious susceptibility to corn and wheat. Ingestion of these two foods had led to mental cloudiness, memory impairment, and other signs of brain-fag.

Her reaction to the oat test was most dramatic, however. This was her last food test in the hospital, made necessary by the fact (initially overlooked) that she ate oats in some form almost every day: oatmeal porridge, oatmeal cookies, and so forth. After twenty minutes, the test seemed to be negative, and I left the hospital. Miss Tolliver, however, went into a severe reaction to the oats, as was revealed when a nurse's assistant came into her room and made an innocent comment. Miss Tolliver misinterpreted the comment and became very annoyed; she insisted that the nurse apologize and angrily started calling all over the hospital, demanding to be discharged and cursing out the administrators. It was only in retrospect that she realized that her reaction was, indeed, a cerebral reaction to a common food eaten with addictive regularity—the oats. In fact, this sort of violent moodiness was familiar to her from previous reactions. Avoidance of her incriminated foods, particularly the three grains mentioned, led to an increase in her mental acuity. She eventually found and kept another job.

When brain-fag was first diagnosed, it was believed that food allergy was the sole cause. After 1950, clinical ecologists became aware of the importance of the chemical environment to health. Cases began to be seen which were primarily caused by exposure to common environmental chemicals.

CASE STUDY: BRAIN-FAG WITH CHEMICAL SUSCEPTIBILITY

Beverly Mehta came to me after reading in a popular sports weekly about my treatment of golf professional Billy Caspar. Miss Mehta was a singer and a teacher, but multiple, unexplained health problems were interfering with both of these activities. She often ran a low-grade fever of undetermined origin. She had rhinitis (runny nose). Above all, she suffered from physical and mental exhaustion and seemed to be unable to rouse herself to do anything. Because of the severity of her symptoms, she was hospitalized for diagnosis.

On the first day of her fast, a terrible headache set in. Her eyes became highly sensitive to light. On the next day she was listless, tired, and nauseated most of the time. Her head and legs ached. On the third day of the fast the symptoms started to clear. By the end of her five-day fast, she was feeling quite well—better than she had in a long time, she said.

Many foods, even in their chemically less contaminated form, caused unexpected symptoms. For example, lobster was followed by a hot, gassy sensation in her stomach. Her ears and eyes hurt, and two-and-a-half hours later her eyes were still visibly red, her glands swollen and painful.

Eating an orange was followed by a ringing sensation in the ears (tinnitus), itching, and chest pains. Carrots were associated with belching and sighing respiration. Potatoes made her feel hot and nauseous, with tremendous itching, perspiration, and sore throat. Her face became red and blotchy.

Wheat induced an equally dramatic reaction. First Miss Mehta felt warm and got transient pains in her fingers. She started sighing and complained that she felt as if "someone had given me knockout drops." She said that she felt like crying, but couldn't. These cerebral reactions were accompanied by belching, nausea, and coughing—and all this from some "innocent" wheat.

Coffee brought on "weepy" feelings. Corn and corn sugar caused a jump in her pulse rate from 90 to 135 beats per minute, a finding which Dr. Arthur Coca believed indicates food allergy.[3]

There were other foods to which Miss Mehta had no reactions. When some of these were given to her in a chemically more contaminated form, however, she had equally dramatic responses. Canned peaches were followed by huskiness in her voice and a chilled feeling which required her to be brought extra robes and blankets. She developed a sore throat, and her temperature rose to 100°F. "This is the way I feel at home much of the time," said the young musician. "I simply sit in front of the television, with little desire to do anything. When I'm singing I slur my words at times like this."

Athought she left the hospital in good condition, when she returned home she soon became sick again, with many of the brain-fag symptoms, although she had tried to follow the prescribed regimen. She told of feeling even worse at work.

I therefore decided to make a house call and I inspected her house and her place of employment for environmental sources of reactions. Her classroom was in the basement of a church. The janitor cheerfully showed me the plethora of chemicals used to clean the premises and to spray for insects on a regular basis. As I entered the room, I was immediately struck by the odor of solvent. The children in Miss Mehta's class sat around a low table with big pads in front of them. Each child held an oversize marking pen of the solvent-based kind in his hand. The fumes from the pens filled the air. I also detected the odor of petroleum candles coming in from the church above. I suggested to Miss Mehta that this environment was helping to perpetuate her brain-fag symptoms and that she seek another job, which she did.

I did not hear from her for a number of years. Then one day she called: she had gone back to college, then to medical school, and was doing well. But she had gotten into the habit of drinking ten cups of coffee a day to keep up with the grueling amount of work. I helped her break this addiction. She finally graduated and became a physician.

This case illustrates very well most of the features of environmental disease. The patient did not have just one or two neatly defined symptoms, but many and varied complaints, physical and allegedly mental. Because of this, other doctors tended to dismiss her problem as "hysterical" in origin. The actual illness remained hidden from Miss Mehta, as it did from her physicians, because of nature's own coverup of food and chemical susceptibility. It was only through the methods of clinical ecology that her many symptoms could be put into some recognizable framework (the plusses and minuses) and her particular problem could be worked out.

It turned out in this case, as in every other, that the particular causes of illness were *unique* for this teacher, just as they are unique for every allergic patient. There was no universal prescription or panacea for *all* such cases, no pill, potion, or drug which could really serve as a cure-all.

Beverly Mehta was fortunate in that her allergy was discovered and corrected, and she went on to have a useful and productive life. Many others have seen their ecologic illness progress to the final stage, the minus-four category.

In summary, one of the most commonly occurring symptoms in medicine, and especially in the histories of allergy patients, is chronic fatigue. Although fatigue may be the only manifestation of clinical ecology, it more commonly exists in conjunction with other manifestations. It occurs so frequently with brain-fag—especially among students—that the two conditions are best described together. Indeed, this combination is often a cause of students being accused of not working up to their measured expectations.[4]

15
Depression (Minus-three and Minus-four Reactions)

For millions of people, depression is a living hell. Traditionally associated with middle or old age, it also afflicts young people as well. Depression can ruin childhood, blight marriage, destroy careers, and wreck plans for a happy retirement. Indirectly, depression can kill, since it is responsible for many of the suicides in our country. Depression is marked by lethargy, disorientation, melancholy, and/or unresponsiveness. The depressed person is usually rational, but can lapse into paranoid or deluded thinking.

Few medical problems are as difficult to treat as depression. A number of procedures have been developed, such as electroshock therapy, psychotherapy, and drug therapy. There is no need here to dissect the successes and failures of these established methods. Each of them has had its vogue, and new drug therapies (such as lithium chloride for manic-depressive disease) come along periodically. What many of them have in common, however, is a *symptomatic* approach. They attempt to relieve the results of the disease, rather than discovering and eliminating the underlying environmental factors which are responsible.

The treatment of depression by the methods of clinical ecology has been successful, on the other hand, because it concentrates on discovering causative factors. As with other manifestations of allergy, the responsible exposures lie in the physical and chemical environment of the patient. This would seem to be the most obvious place to look for the source of an illness, yet most doctors never consider the actual, material surroundings at all. It is easier and more lucrative to treat symptoms.

Depression can be either a minus-three or a minus-four symptom, depending on the degree of severity. It is the end of the line for many individuals who are maladapted to their environment. Depression rarely strikes out of the blue.

147

It is preceded, in most cases, by a prolonged period of illness, including both stimulatory reactions and lesser withdrawal reactions.

In fact, the alternation of extreme stimulatory symptoms (mania) and extreme withdrawal symptoms (depression) is well recognized in the medical literature as "manic-depressive disease." In this illness, the patient's mood changes from "highs" to "lows" quite rapidly. There is an ever-increasing tendency, however, for the "down" periods to crowd out the "up" periods. Depression becomes more and more the rule, while the overexcited manic phase becomes less frequent and less prolonged. While this disease is recognized in its most extreme form, doctors generally fail to see the alternation of stimulatory and withdrawal symptoms in less advanced cases.

Both depression and manic-depressive disease can be the result of environmental factors such as commonly eaten foods and chemicals. The two illnesses can occur alone but more commonly are found in conjunction with a long list of other symptoms in susceptible persons.

It has long been suspected that some persons are depressed because of reactions to nonpersonal environmental exposures. My first demonstration of this was a motion picture filmed in 1950[1] and reported preliminarily.[2] Hydrocarbon exposures were demonstrated as causes of depression in 1956.[3] Confirmation and extension of these observations of the effects of given foods in highly susceptible persons led to a scientific exhibit at the Annual Meeting of the American Psychiatric Association in 1956 and the founding of the Section on Allergy of the Nervous System of the American College of Allergists in 1957. This was called ecologic mental illness in 1959.[4] Numerous subsequent reports are listed in a bibliography, which will be provided upon request, as mentioned earlier.

Others, especially Donan and associates,[5,6] Speer,[7] Mackarness,[8,10] Mandell and Scanlon,[9] and Philpott and Kalita,[11] have published in this area.

It so happened that these observations of the causative demonstrable roles of foods and environmental chemicals in depression and related mental illnesses were first noted in 1950, the same year that psychotrophic drugs became available to physicians. Since these mass-applicable approaches were promoted vigorously by their manufacturers, the highly individualized approaches of clinical ecology did not receive serious trials for several years until the hazards associated with psychotrophic drugs became more apparent.

CASE STUDY: DEPRESSION WITH HEADACHE

Meryl Avery suffered from depression, with occasional seizures of panic, for six years. Before that she had had a long history of physical and mental-like problems, although she was still in her twenties.

As a baby she had thrown up easily, and she had wet her bed until she was fourteen. As a child, she would sometimes hold her breath until she turned blue in the face and passed out. She had many mysterious "infections." By the time she entered college, however, she seemed to be doing fairly well.

The long drive home from college during her freshman year triggered her ill health once again, however. She became acutely ill during the trip, and when she reached home, she could not walk but had to *crawl* up the stairs to her bedroom, crying all the way. She had a severe headache, was sick all night, and had residual symptoms on the following day.

The other passengers in the car also got headaches, but only Meryl became so desperately sick. In retrospect, her friends figured that there was a leak in the exhaust system of the car and that some of the fumes and carbon monoxide had gotten into the passenger compartment. None of the passengers could recall smelling any exhaust odors, however, or noticing anything unusual about the trip. The car was checked out and was not found to be defective.

While the other people recovered, Meryl's health started a precipitous decline. She was plagued by weakness, fatigue, and dizziness at school. She started getting headaches again, a problem she had had frequently as a teenager. She took stimulatory drugs—"White Crosses," or "uppers"—and alcohol to relieve feelings of weakness and mental exhaustion.

Because of these problems she was unable to attend most of her classes and lost credit for the term. The trip home was again traumatic, and she arrived in tears. To be closer to home, Meryl transferred to another college, but her problems became worse. She cried almost continually, threw temper tantrums, and was soon depressed most of the time. Her eating habits deteriorated: she practically lived on "instant breakfasts."

Her reading comprehension declined. Her memory was poor; she was unable to handle taxing situations and "froze up" on examinations. During the next summer she visited relatives in the rural South and, simultaneously, contacted a nutritionist who was familiar with clinical ecology. The combination of relatively pure air and a partial diagnosis of her food problem worked wonders. "I discovered what it was like to feel good," she later said in reference to this time. For the next six months she remained on a Rotary Diversified Diet and avoided some incriminated foods. But on Christmas day, at a family party, she began cheating on this diet and continued to slip downhill all week. The binge ended in a marathon cookie-eating session, in a room with a gas fireplace.

The next morning Meryl was, as she says, "totally freaked out." Although she kept taking alkali salts, which can often ameliorate allergic symptoms, and ate what she thought were her compatible foods, she could not regain her previous feelings of health. She screamed and hit the walls, the furniture took on odd shapes, and she became severely depressed. Her sister had to come and calm her down.

Finally, she sought help at the Ecology Unit. After an initial period of headaches and itchy eyes, she felt well again. She reacted to several of the waters tested, but one was found with which she was compatible.

The worst reactions were as follows: Eating corn was followed by blotchy face and itchiness; cod brought hot feelings, tingling in the neck and shoulders, panic which came on quickly, and headache. Red snapper brought severe depression, crying, panic, and a "spacey" feeling. Eggs were followed by aches and pains all over and panic after two hours. After eating rabbit she fell asleep and then awoke in panic, crying and depressed. Avocado brought sleepiness, after which she awoke depressed and angry. Cauliflower was accompanied by an immediate depression. Between such tests, or when given compatible foods, she was pleasant and cheerful.

We next took some of Meryl's safe foods and fed them to her in their chemically contaminated form, just as they came from the supermarket, presumably contaminated with residues of pesticides and preservatives. Within ninety minutes of her first meal, she developed a severe depression which lasted for several hours.

Food reactions are not always traceable to *commonly* eaten foods. Often a person will react, or rather cross-react, to less frequently eaten foods, if those foods "remind" the body of other, allergy-causing substances. In Meryl's case, however, there was a clear link between her reactions and her eating habits.

She had previously reported a craving for sweets and a severe reaction to cookies. These usually contained corn syrup, and thus it is not surprising that she had a strong reaction to corn and corn sugar in her hospital diagnostic test. People with such allergies, as explained in Chapter 10, also frequently are allergic to alcoholic beverages, which often contain corn in some form. Meryl had reported severe reactions to alcoholic beverages of all sorts and was on the verge of becoming an alcoholic. She had a serious reaction in the hospital to yeast, which is an ingredient in all alcoholic beverages. After the nutritionist had diagnosed some of Meryl's food allergies, she had switched to fish as a supposedly safe food, but she had eaten it in an addictive way, having it for breakfast every day. Thus it is not surprising that she should have had very severe reactions to cod and red snapper.

Many of Meryl's problems seemed in retrospect to have been related to her chemical-susceptibility problem (which was demonstrated by her reaction to contaminated food). Her initial experience returning from college was probably related to car exhaust fumes. These could have been relatively "normal" amounts of exhausts which often seep into cars traveling at highway speeds. The other people in the car were apparently less susceptible to this influence, and suffered either transient headaches or no symptoms at all. By adhering to a new diet, and minimizing her exposure to chemical pollution, Meryl was able to finish college and begin a successful career.

CASE STUDY: DEPRESSION WITH FATIGUE AND OBESITY

Francine Phillips was a graduate student who had been periodically depressed and fatigued since high school. Basically intelligent and capable, she often had periods in which she could not perform even simple tasks. She also suffered from obesity.

She herself suspected that "sugar" was the cause of her problem (most people do not differentiate between the various forms of sugar). She believed, as well, that part of her weight problem was caused by fluid retention. She reported feeling swollen after eating a heavy meal. She said that she could gain three or four pounds in a day, but that she could also lose ten pounds on a crash diet. Miss Phillips also suspected that she was allergic to certain kinds of water and reported abdominal bloating whenever she drank tap water.

When she was treated in the Ecology Unit, her depression became worse before it gradually lessened. At the end of the fast period, she felt well. She was then tested on various waters, and she did, in fact, react to several of them, including chlorinated city water.

Her own suspicions about foods were largely correct. She reacted with depression, headache, or fatigue to corn and corn sugar and also to cane sugar, as well as to tea and coffee. She also had lesser reactions to onions, acorn squash, walnuts, lettuce, potatoes, chocolate, and honey.

She also reacted to some foods tolerated in their organic form when she was fed them in their commercial, supermarket form. This was taken as a positive test for chemical susceptibility.

Miss Phillips' case was not very advanced, and her depression was rated at a minus-three level. With careful control of food intake and avoidance of environmental chemicals (Chap. 20), she has been able to lead a happier life and pursue her studies without interruption.

CASE STUDY: DEPRESSION AND OBESITY

A similar, but much more serious case was presented by Eleanor Wyckham, an overweight middle-aged woman. Two years before entering the Ecology Unit, Mrs. Wyckham had been hospitalized for depression. She had attempted suicide twice and had been given electroshock therapy. In her case, the treatment was ineffective and caused some memory loss.

Mrs. Wyckham was one of those patients who was aware that her problems stemmed in part from food. "I've reached the point where I am afraid to eat any longer," she said, before entering the Ecology Unit. "Once I start eating, I feel as if I simply cannot stop." She alternated between binges of eating and fasts or all-fruit diets. Her favorite food in the world, she said, was peanut butter—this was the one item she could not do without. She also loved bread, baked goods, and in fact anything with wheat in it. She had eaten wheat addictively since childhood, when her mother, who was interested in nutrition, became convinced of the virtues of whole wheat bread. She therefore plied her daughter with large amounts of this staple. Mrs. Wyckham, who had a family history of alcoholism, likened herself to an alcoholic, too—in her craving for bread and peanut butter.

She entered the hospital in a very depressed state. After five days of fasting, she was much less depressed. Not surprisingly, in her food test she had a severe reaction to peanuts (as well as to lamb). More unexpected was the fact that she passed the wheat test with no trouble—which shows that food allergies cannot always be pinpointed on the basis of histories or "hunches." She did have moderate reactions to yeast and milk, however, which are often components of bread.

Mrs. Wyckham was then retested on some of the foods to which she had had no adverse reaction, but this time to foods which had been purchased in a commercial market. There was a definite increase in her depression, after a few such meals. Through the avoidance of incriminated foods, Mrs. Wyckham was able to control both her depression and her weight problem. This points to the fact that the Rotary Diversified Diet (Chap. 18), although not specifically designed as a weight-loss diet, can be helpful in that regard for the overweight patient.

The patients described in the preceding cases appear to have become sicker gradually, after a long period of cumulative exposure to chemicals and foods. Sometimes, however, a preexisting condition is suddenly made much worse by a massive exposure to an allergy-causing substance.

CASE STUDY: DEPRESSION WITH FATIGUE

Connie Mullens was an attractive woman in her early thirties. She appeared to have many of the things which would help to make a person happy: a loving spouse, a beautiful home, a good educational background, and a rewarding job. Yet before she came to the Ecology Unit, she was contemplating suicide. Mrs. Mullens had many illnesses and problems practically all her life, but was completely unhelped by conventional treatment. In fact, her health was endangered by being prescribed amphetamines. Clinical ecology helped her, in part by breaking her dependence on these drugs.

During her childhood, she had had many illnesses, some of them bizarre. She had had asthma so badly that her parents doubted at times that she would live. This problem went away after the family moved to a new house. In high school, she had frequent stomach problems, diagnosed as the result of a "virus." One such "virus" lasted for over a year.

In college, she demonstrated superior academic ability, got straight A's most of the time, and was elected to Phi Beta Kappa. Nevertheless, during this same period a curious sort of malaise started to creep over her, imperceptibly at first.

At times, especially in chemistry lab, she would feel a kind of euphoria. She was known as the chemistry class prankster and would devise complicated practical jokes to play on her instructors. Of course, this sort of behavior among college students is "normal" when looked at in isolation. It is only when seen in the context of her overall development, and the onset of her more serious symptoms, that it begins to take on medical significance. In retrospect, some of this behavior may have been a lesser stimulatory reaction (plus-one) to the presence of chemicals and natural gas (in the bunsen burners) in the classroom.

At the same time, Mrs. Mullens had an increasing number of bad days. On these occasions, she had headaches of ever-increasing frequency and intensity. On some days, she could not get out of bed, could not concentrate, and could barely stay awake. To combat these doldrums, she relied on junk food. She would drink cola beverages or eat chocolate and candy whenever she had to "cram" for a test. Every day she would go down to the drugstore and have a chocolate malt and a piece of pie, which seemed to temporarily relieve her tiredness and headaches.

Because she was, not surprisingly, overweight, she consulted an internist, who prescribed diet pills which contained amphetamines. "With these," she later recalled, "I could leap tall buildings at a single bound." She stopped taking them when she realized that she was becoming addicted.

Connie was married in college, but the marriage did not work out. This was mainly because of her irritability, she says. She would throw temper tantrums in the house, fling shoes at her husband, or force him to watch his favorite television shows with the sound off (she was very sensitive to noise). She kept on eating, too; her husband called her the "cookie monster" because of her insatiable sweet tooth.

By the time she reached graduate school, her problems were worse. She now had headaches once or twice a week, but each lasted a couple of days. She began to consult doctors, and each had a different diagnosis and solution. One internist, she says, prescribed twenty different pills, mostly amphetamines. She was instructed to try each of them in turn and keep a record of their effects. None of them did anything for her head pain.

She also saw an endocrinologist (hormone specialist), an otolaryngologist (ear-nose-and-throat specialist), and, of course, a psychiatrist. The psychiatrist analyzed her psyche in depth and at length. He came to the conclusion that, as an only child, she had had too much pressure put on her to achieve. In fact, except for her illnesses, she had had a particularly happy childhood. Her parents were both successful and well-educated and probably expected their daughter to be the same, but did not force her to emulate them in this regard.

Connie could not drive an automobile. If she attempted to she became confused and could not interpret traffic signs or even make sense out of a simple stop light. Rather than look for something in the environment (for example, automobile fumes) that might cause such a condition, the psychiatrist interpreted this problem as a psychological need for perfection. He recommended that she relax more.

After finishing graduate school, Mrs. Mullens undertook a job which brought her into contact with industrial chemicals. All of her symptoms worsened. She got married again and gave up the full-time job.

As bad as all these symptoms were, her condition took a sharp turn for the worse (from minus-two or -three to minus-four) when her new home was sprayed with powerful pesticides, inside and out. Winter came, and the gas-fired heater was turned on. Soon afterward she started to feel so weak that she could not get out of bed. She was depressed to the point of dwelling on suicide. Her new husband would come home each day and find her crying uncontrollably.

Her psychiatrist prescribed amphetamines again, this time for ten days, to bring her out of what he called a "short-term depression." At the end of this period, she was worse and had developed a numbness in her fingers and a tingling in her limbs. To all of her other problems, she now added a fear of multiple sclerosis—an unfounded fear, it now appears.

When she was admitted to the Ecology Unit, her symptoms were particularly bad. The water fast accentuated her symptoms; she developed a terrible headache and cried almost continually at first. After a few days on the fast, however, she underwent a remarkable recovery. "I got completely better," she recalls. "I became absolutely convinced that my problem was related to the environment."

Mrs. Mullens reacted to most of the foods she was given. Some brought on arthritislike aches in her fingers and other joints. The worst food for her was beef. After eating a portion of beef, she told the nurse on duty that she wanted to kill herself. She wandered the halls, crying aimlessly. The next day she said that she felt as if she "had been run over by a bulldozer."

All of her many symptoms were reproduced in several weeks of food testing. What is more, tests with chemicals in various forms showed that this patient had the problem of chemical susceptibility.

Mrs. Mullens has made excellent progress in controlling her food and chemical difficulties. "In the real world we face serious problems," she has said. For example, it is difficult for her to avoid all exposure to natural gas. The gas heater and range have been removed from her house, but she still runs into them in other peoples' homes, as well as in stores. In certain shops, she becomes so irritable that she feels like strangling those who get in her way. It is only in gas-heated stores that she has this problem. Despite periodic setbacks, her mental state recently has been cheerful.

An understanding of the food and chemical problem has brought with it many rewards. But it also has added responsibilities. Once, when she was in a hospital for some physiological testing, a conventional doctor "caught" her making lists of her reactions to artificially colored and flavored medicine. He actually took papers which she had discarded out of the wastebasket, read them, and remarked, "I see that you are involved with your symptoms. You apparently *want* to be sick!" When she tried to reason with the man, who was a gastroenterologist, he said brusquely, "I have forty other cases in the hospital. I don't need you." To his amazement, she promptly checked herself out of the hospital.

Mrs. Mullens' case thus represents both the triumph and the tragedy of treatment by the methods of clinical ecology. On the one hand, like many other patients, she was brought back from the brink of suicide by coming to understand the multiple environmental factors responsible for her reactions. She credits it with saving her life. Yet, on the other hand, the world itself sometimes seems hostile to this new approach. Much yet needs to be done to make the environment completely livable for the Connie Mullenses of this world.

In summary, it may be said that the concepts and techniques of ecologic mental illness are opening up new horizons for patients with the symptoms of depression and related psychiatric disturbances. In contrast to the longstanding artificial distinctions between physical and so-called mental illnesses, both physical and cerebral and behavioral manifestations of allergy/ecology represent different levels of reaction. At long last, large sectors of the field of psychiatry are yielding to medical management based on the demonstrability of cause and effect.

III
COPING WITH THE MODERN ENVIRONMENT

In previous sections, we have looked at the basic concept of clinical ecology and at the different stages and symptoms which environmentally caused disease can engender. In this section, I shall explain in more detail some of the techniques which advocates of this new approach have devised to cope with the ecologic disaster of the twentieth century.

The first problem is one of diagnosis. Conventional medicine recognizes the fact that millions of people are chronically ill and that it can offer little for their arthritis, or migraine, or fatigue, or depression but chemically derived pills. Patients with a welter of confusing symptoms are often treated contemptuously, because the underlying cause of their many illnesses goes unnoticed. By its very nature, the etiology of environmentally caused chronic disease is hidden: this is "nature's medical coverup." The first job of the clinical ecologist is to cut through the confusion and demonstrate the underlying causes with convincing tests.

Over a period of about fifty years, clinical ecologists have worked out procedures which differ from those used by conventional doctors. Even the history-taking interview is different. I practice "poker-faced medicine," in that I do not pass judgment on a patient's symptoms upon first hearing them, no matter how bizarre they may seem. Many such symptoms later turn out to have significance in the patient's medical history. A chemical questionnaire, which is included in Chapter 19, evolved through many editions and helps reveal a patient's susceptibility. The reader can take this test himself and get a preliminary idea of his own degree of sensitivity to chemicals.

Treatment by the methods of clinical ecology is safe, inexpensive, and effective. It is based, primarily, on avoidance of those environmental agents which cause trouble. The Rotary Diversified Diet (described in Chap. 18) works well for all types of food allergies and can help those who wish to diagnose their food allergies, as well as those who wish to avoid their development.

The treatment of chemical susceptibility is also largely based on avoidance. A number of simple and inexpensive procedures are described which can help protect the many people who suffer unknowingly from chemical-related problems.

Taken together, the chapters in this section can help any reader to become more aware of his own highly personalized reaction to common foods and chemicals and to begin to take simple steps to deal with a growing problem.

16
Interviews and In-Office Procedures

The difference between clinical ecology and conventional medicine becomes apparent as soon as one enters the waiting room. In my office, for instance, the physical setup is adjusted to the needs of the susceptible person. This is done to provide a more hospitable environment and also because test procedures undertaken in the office itself might be ruined by chemical exposures.

No smoking is allowed, and this rule is strictly enforced. Signs to this effect are posted not only in the waiting room but in the bathroom as well, where confirmed tobacco addicts may be tempted to depart from the rule. Care has been taken in the selection of office furniture. Wood and leather are used extensively, not plastic or synthetics. Office machinery is kept to a minimum in order to avoid the kinds of fumes and odors which frequently foul the air indoors. Almost all of the typewriters, for instance, are manual, not electric. The copying machine was chosen because it emits the least amount of environmental pollutants. In fact, it is rarely used. Even the partitions are made of hardwood and not of any building material which gives off gases, as plastics often do. Nurses, secretaries, and other employees are instructed to refrain not only from smoking but also from the use of perfumes, scents, and after-shave lotions. We have little trouble in this regard, however, for almost all office personnel themselves have food and chemical susceptibilities, and are chosen with this fact in mind. Because of their own experience, they can provide more help and understanding to patients than those who are not aware of environmental disease in a personal way.

The office is located high above Lake Michigan, and the air is about as good as one is likely to find in a big city like Chicago. For heat, we employ portable electric heaters. In a sense, then, a patient's treatment begins as soon as he enters the office itself, since the environment is conducive to recovery.

Taking the Medical History

The taking of a medical history also reveals the difference between ours and the traditional approach. Traditional medicine is centered on the body and its various organs. It is called *anthropocentric*, or *body-centered*, medicine. A traditional doctor is mainly concerned with treating the body and focusing primarily upon the most distressing physical symptom or "chief complaint."

In the traditional history, previous medical problems will also be noted briefly, but in general there is no attempt to link seemingly unrelated "nonmedical," past problems in the patient's life to the present illness. Of course not— for no theoretical framework exists to make such connections. In general, symptoms and organs are neatly compartmentalized and viewed in relative isolation from one another. The history of a person's illness is thus seen narrowly, as the history of one particular symptom or syndrome, rather than broadly, as a history of increasing ill health stemming from environmental exposures.

Although the dates of important medical changes may be indicated on the record, the reader of such a traditional medical history tends to be relatively unaware of the long-term progression of symptoms which may have preceded the current illness. In addition, traditional medical histories tell almost nothing about the environmental facts of a patient's life. The doctor rarely asks about the details of job or hobby, about cooking or heating systems in the home, or methods of insect control used in the patient's vicinity. To him, these seem irrelevant and outside the practice of medicine as he was taught it in medical school.

If currently available tests show no "organic" disease, the doctor is more likely to ask probing (and sometimes leading) questions about interpersonal relationships, such as problems with a spouse, children, or parents. Generally speaking, however, little effort is made to relate the "chief complaint" to other problems in the patient's life, and the "medical" facts tend to be separated from the environmental facts.

The basic cause of a chronic illness is rarely exposed by this type of traditional history-taking. Since the doctor fails to comprehend the subtle and hidden give-and-take between the environment and the patient, with its ever-shifting balance of environmental challenge and individual response, he cannot understand the patient's seemingly unclassifiable illness.

A patient with a long history and a thick file frequently becomes a "neurotic" in the doctor's eyes, and this judgment is passed along from one doctor to another. In such an atmosphere, doctors tend to become cynical about many patients' complaints, while patients bitterly reject established medicine.

I call this traditional approach the "ABCDs of modern mass-applicable medicine." A stands for *Analytical:* the medical profession tends to chop problems up into neatly compartmentalized specialties, rather than seeing the broad outlines in a *synthesized* (unifying) fashion. *B* and *C*, in this scheme, stand for *Body-Centered.* The doctor looks at the body but fails to see the environment (mainly physical and nonpersonal) which impinges on that body at every step and with every breath. *D* stands for *Drug-oriented.* The traditional physician almost always uses drugs to alter or neutralize symptoms whose basic cause(s) he does not understand. Analytical, Body-Centered, Drug-oriented medicine has many achievements to its credit, but it offers little to the growing number of patients who are suffering from environmentally induced chronic illness.

The history-taking of clinical ecologists is quite different. Whereas in traditional medicine, the taking of the history (which is one of the most important portions of the diagnostic process) is usually assigned to the *least* experienced member of the medical team (the intern or medical student), the clinical ecologist himself usually conducts his own interviews. Some people think a doctor wastes valuable time by doing this. If important leads are to be uncovered, however, it is necessary for one experienced person to be familiar with the details of each individual case.

Because of the essentially addictive nature of many environmental problems, especially in their earlier, or stimulatory, phases, medical histories can be paradoxically misleading. For example, an untrained history-taker can overlook the significance of a patient's remark that he "loves" or "craves" a particular food or chemical, and that eating, drinking, or inhaling that item makes him feel better. A conventionally trained doctor or nurse is likely to encourage the patient in the use of such a substance, while a clinical ecologist will immediately suspect it as a source of allergic/addictive responses.

The form of the interview which a clinical ecologist conducts is also different from that in traditional, ABCD medicine. Instead of looking at the body as a collection of various organs and parts, with medical and scientific subspecialties organized to deal with isolated problems which affect them, clinical ecology emphasizes the *wholeness* of the individual and the uniqueness of his experience. It thus forms part of the larger movement toward "holistic" medicine, which is gaining increasing importance.

Emphasis is put on recording events in a chronological fashion. The patient's illness must be traced not just to the onset of the present symptom but to the beginning of his overall ill health. This, in turn, must be correlated with significant events in his life history.

Getting the medical history usually takes me about one hour. First, I generally let the patient explain who referred him and why he has come, in his own terms. If he has come because of a well-defined problem, such as headache, I ask him when he started having headaches and let him make any statement he wishes about this problem.

If the patient cannot single out any overriding problem but simply feels chronically ill, with many complaints, I ask him when he ceased being well and started feeling poorly. In other words, I try to orient the history (as the name implies) to the *development* of the problem *in time.* However, some people cannot give a chronological history. Either they do not think in those terms or their minds are too clouded by their disease. In these cases, I simply ask the patient to state all of his symptoms according to the categories explained in Chapter 8. Briefly, the categories are: *physical localized symptoms: 1)* upper respiratory, *2)* lower respiratory, *3)* gastrointestinal, *4)* dermatological, *5)* genitourinary. *Physical systemic symptoms: 1)* fatigue, *2)* headache, *3)* myalgia, *4)* arthralgia. *Mental-behavioral symptoms: a)* brain-fag *b)* depression, with or without altered consciousness.

I gather in the data, typing whatever the patient says, without making off-hand interpretations. After about an hour, good clues usually emerge from this narrative, although the cause of the illness cannot be known for certain until actual testing is done.

The medical history is supplemented with forms and tests, such as the Chemical Questionnaire reprinted in Chapter 19. On the basis of the results of the interview, questionnaires, and tests, the patient is then assigned to one of two groups. One group, constituting about half of my referred practice, are patients who are so seriously ill that they must be hospitalized to undergo further testing and treatment. The method of helping such patients is explained in the following chapters. The less severely afflicted, or those who are unable to be hospitalized for a variety of reasons, are diagnosed and treated on an in-office (outpatient) basis.

Testing for Food Allergies

In the office, we use what are called *provocative tests* to detect food allergies. This is an excellent technique, although not quite as reliable or convincing as the food ingestion tests employed in the hospital. These provocative tests provide reactions in miniature, as it were, between four and thirty minutes after their application.

The tests are called provocative, since they seek to *provoke* a response in the patient to a suspected food. Clinical ecologists maintain a large number of extracts of various substances. If, in his history, the patient indicates exposures to any food once every three days or more frequently, or if he himself suspects a particular one, he will be tested with a drop of an extract of it placed under his tongue. Generally, the patient can complete two such tests on each visit, until he has tested all of the foods which he most commonly encounters. If a reaction is severe, however, only one test will be given.

As with a number of other innovations in this field, the provocative test was discovered by a doctor who himself had allergies he wished to control. Dr. Carleton Lee, of St. Joseph, Missouri, was highly susceptible to coffee. In the early 1960s, Lee found that he was able to create his characteristic coffee "hangover" with a minute intradermal (skin-deep) injection of coffee extract. In other words, he "provoked" the symptoms with a small dose. Even more intriguing was the fact that a still smaller dose would relieve the same symptoms and keep them in check for hours or days, even when he then drank coffee freely. He called this latter injection the "neutralizing" dose.

Intradermal injections for food allergies had been tried before but with little consistent success. For inhaled allergy-causing substances, such as pollen and dust, they had worked well, but for foods and chemicals they had never been very valuable. Lee presented his findings to food-allergy pioneer Herbert Rinkel, and together they published the first paper on the provocative/neutralizing technique in January, 1962.[1]

Dr. Guy Pfeiffer and Dr. Lawrence D. Dickey soon refined Lee's intradermal test by making it a sublingual (under-the-tongue) procedure. The veins under the tongue are close to the surface and readily absorb traces of foods, beverages, and drugs. (It is for this reason that nitroglycerine and some other drugs are placed under the tongue for immediate absorption.) Sublingual extracts worked approximately as well as intradermal injections and avoided the unpleasantness of the injections. Both techniques are currently employed by clinical ecologists, although I myself prefer, and actually use, the sublingual provocative test in my office procedures.

Why the provocative/neutralizing technique works, we do not yet know. That it does work has been demonstrated in hundreds of physicians' offices, although some orthodox allergists committed to the immunological theory remain skeptical. The provocative/neutralizing technique is a truly empirical procedure, used because it has been found to be effective. If we were to wait until the mechanism of every medical procedure were known before being used, few drugs, new or old, could be employed in medicine. Even the mechanism by which aspirin works is still something of a mystery, and the action of electroshock and tricyclic drugs for depression still must be accounted for. The provocative/neutralizing technique can be used in the same spirit, while research is performed on its mechanism of action.

After performing a provocative test with an extract of a commonly eaten food, we are likely to provoke a positive reaction. In about nine out of ten cases, the patient will respond with the same symptoms which the food is secretly responsible for in real life. If wheat, for example, is the hidden cause of respiratory symptoms, the patient might respond by suddenly coughing or wheezing. Sometimes, however, the symptoms provoked are one notch worse than the real-life symptoms. Thus, a patient who gets headaches (minus-two symptom) from cane sugar under normal conditions might become depressed (minus-three) or brain-fagged (minus-three) after a provocative test with cane.

Once a troublesome reaction has been provoked in this manner, we then attempt to find a neutralizing dose of the same substance. The purpose of this, in our office, is to spare the patient from having to go home with aggravated symptoms. This is the only use to which I generally put the neutralizing technique. Some doctors use the neutralizing dose as a regular *treatment* for food and chemical susceptibilities, however, providing the patient with a vial of extract to take on a daily or interim basis.

I generally do not do this, since the majority of my patients come to me from out of town. The dose frequently needs readjusting, as, for example, during hay-fever season, at times of virus infection, or for other reasons. It does little good for a patient to call me and say, "Doctor, my dose is no longer working," when he lives five hundred or a thousand miles from Chicago. I generally help such patients to find a doctor nearer home who will provide such treatments: a list of such clinical ecologists can be obtained from the Society for Clinical Ecology, whose address is listed in Appendix C.

Clinical ecologists, it should be noted, do not generally use the familiar scratch or skin tests employed by most conventional allergists, since they do not give definitive results. According to Albert Rowe, M.D., "It is generally agreed that clinical allergy may exist in the absence of positive skin reactions, especially those to the scratch test. This is true primarily in food allergy and to a lesser extent in inhalant allergy."[2] In a statistical study of intradermal skin tests, Rinkel found such tests to be only forty percent accurate, and often less so.[3]

Chemical Susceptibility and In-Office Treatment

Lee and Rinkel originally devised the provocative/neutralizing dose for the diagnosis and treatment of food allergies. It still remained necessary to devise such a test for the in-office diagnosis and treatment of the chemical-susceptibility problem. This test was a by-product of the alcoholism studies which I made, described in Chapter 10. In the course of those studies, a batch of pure, 100-proof synthetic ethyl alcohol was obtained, derived from a petrochemical, ethylene gas. This type of alcohol, although not approved for drinking, is found in various food products, such as lemon and orange extracts. It is not toxic per se.

When given to chemically susceptible individuals, however, it can provoke reactions similar to those they experienced from environmental chemical exposures. The synthetic alcohol was mixed in graded dilutions. Dilution no. 1 was 1:5 mixture of ethyl alcohol and a salt solution; no. 2 was in a proportion of 1:25 (that is, one-fifth as strong as no. 1); and so forth.

If a patient answered at least two questions positively on the Chemical Questionnaire he was tested with a few drops of dilution no. 2, either by injection intradermally or under the tongue. If he answered three to five questions positively, he was tested with dilution no. 3; greater degrees of susceptibility were treated with even weaker dilutions.

In this way, it was possible to test patients for this perplexing chemical-susceptibility problem in the office and to receive fairly reliable results quickly. Before that, a patient had to move out of his house for a while to get such an answer, whereas today the best tests are performed in the hospital (Chapter 17). I published, preliminarily, the results of this test in 1964.[4]

Using this same synthetic ethyl alcohol as a neutralizing dose, it was possible to relieve the symptoms of some patients for a long period of time. The technique was used especially on those who could not avoid chemical exposure, either because of their jobs, the location of their homes, or for other reasons.

One patient, for example, was a domestic maid who had to travel more than five miles by bus every day, five times a week. Each day she would get a headache on the bus, often before she had even reached her destination. She was provided with a small bottle of ethyl alcohol, at the dilution which had previously been found to suit her. By taking a drop of the solution under her tongue, she was able to relieve her headaches.

Another woman lived on the edge of a golf course. Because of continual pesticide spraying, she was chronically ill. After learning to use a neutralizing dose of the synthetic ethyl alcohol, however, she was not only able to tolerate life in her home, but was even able to play golf on the course without suffering any health problems. Because both ethyl alcohol and the pesticides are ultimately derived from the same substances—petrochemicals—a neutralizing dose made of one substance can have an effect in relieving symptoms caused by another such substance.

This is not meant to imply that such drops are a kind of cure-all for the chemical-susceptibility problem. Unfortunately, they are not. Such treatments are not fully protective, because a person's intake of chemicals varies greatly with time and place.

In addition to synthetic ethyl alcohol, various other chemical extracts now aid in the treatment of chemically susceptible patients. One of the most ingenious is an extract of automobile fumes which Dr. Harris Hosen of Port Arthur, Texas, prepared for the use of clinical ecologists.[5] This is sometimes quite effective in detecting and relieving the effects of smog and the fumes of heavy traffic on susceptible patients.

Basically, however, the most effective "treatment" devised for the chemically susceptible patient is still prevention. In Chapter 20, some steps which the reader can take to prevent the occurrence and spread of this modern plague are described.

It should be reemphasized that patients with advanced environmentally related illness involving food and chemicals are also often sensitive to pollens, molds, dusts, animal danders, insect emanations, and other inhaled particles. Indeed, the course of environmentally related events often starts with localized allergic manifestations on such a basis. But, as Dr. Mandell has emphasized, pollens, molds, etc., may also be related causally to advanced systemic or generalized effects.[6] Since skin testing with extracts of these materials is relatively reliable, this possibility should be evaluated by measuring the degree of skin sensitivity as a basis for providing optimal injection therapy.

17
The Ecology Unit

The Ecology Unit (sometimes referred to as the Environmental Control Unit) plays an indispensable role in the diagnosis and treatment of allergies. This unit was established after many years of development.

I first started hospitalizing patients for the diagnosis of food allergy in 1950. I chose complicated patients, whose problems could not be worked out simply by testing with one food at a time in the office. (In those days I employed feedings of whole foods in the office, rather than provocative tests, as today.) These patients rarely ever achieved a "base line" of good health before any particular test against which their reaction could be measured. It was therefore impossible to tell to what extent a particular food, or other environmental exposure, was responsible for their symptoms.

At this same time, I had occasion to present some of my earliest patients with "mental" symptoms to the psychiatrists at the Milwaukee Sanitorium. Dr. Josef Kindwall, chief of staff at this well-respected institution, listened to my presentation and then suggested that I *fast* such patients, in order to clear the board, so to speak, of all preexisting symptoms.

Six patients were therefore hospitalized in separate rooms and fasted. Each patient soon complained of *heightened* symptoms and, being inexperienced, I was disturbed by their worsened condition and decided to cancel the tests. In fact, these heightened symptoms in the early part of a fast are now known to be normal *withdrawal* reactions to addicting foods. Thus the initial attempt to fast patients ended in failure.

In April, 1951, the chemical-susceptibility problem was first described, and so, in the winter of 1953, were the effects of natural gas on susceptible individuals (Chapter 6). Considering these unexpected sources of reactions, it became even more obvious that in order to achieve a "base line" of health, it would be necessary to remove a patient to a sheltered environment, in which food and chemical exposures could be thoroughly controlled. This belief was reinforced by seeing an occasional patient who felt distinctly better in the chemically less contaminated environment of a hospital. Some doctors referred to this phenomenon as "hospitalitis," an alleged "disease" in which an individual craves a protective environment, but I believed the reason lay in the effects of the nonpersonal environment on the patient's health.

In the meantime, I told Dr. Donald S. Mitchell of Montreal about my difficulties in fasting patients and about the need to do so, given the complexity of their problems. Dr. Mitchell, on his own initiative, attempted to confirm this and was able to fast patients for longer periods of time. He discovered that the withdrawal symptoms subsided by the third or fourth day and that after that, the patients generally felt better than they had in a long while.

In 1956, I therefore decided to attempt a hospital fasting program again. This time the experiment was a success, and certain food and chemical allergies were diagnosed which simply could not have been found through any of the office procedures used at that time.

This experience led to a new approach to the diagnosis of allergy-caused illnesses. Since that time, I have hospitalized, fasted, and tested over 10,000 individuals in this manner. Until 1975, such testing was done in separate hospital rooms of a general hospital. Patients did reasonably well in this environment. One problem, however, was that chemically susceptible patients were still exposed to tobacco smoke, perfumes, and other hospital fumes and odors, which interfered with the accuracy and validity of the testing. Sometimes night nurses might smoke in the nursing stations. At other times rooms were chemically disinfected and residues of such agents made certain rooms unavailable for use.

Since 1975, therefore, a separate Ecology Unit has been maintained as a section of a hospital in a Chicago suburb, and it is far more controlled than any ordinary hospital room or ward could be.[1]

The procedures in the Ecology Unit are an indispensable part of the treatment for allergy. Traditional diagnostic techniques are like a table with three legs. The first leg is the patient's history, the second his physical examination, and the third his diagnostic tests. In the Ecology Unit, all three of these standard methods are employed, but in addition there is a fourth leg. Often it is this fourth diagnostic leg which provides the sound basis for an answer. Its value has been confirmed by many physicians, and about a dozen are now using this sort of hospitalization in their daily practice. Indeed, in the combined experience of clinical ecologists using these techniques in a hospital or environmentally controlled setting, approximately 20,000 patients have been observed under controlled conditions during the past three decades (see Appendix B for a list of clinical ecologists practicing in a controlled environmental hospital setting).

The basic idea of the Ecology Unit is *control*. For several weeks, all aspects of the patient's physical environment are scientifically managed. The air he breathes, the food and water he consumes, and everything that might come into contact with, or enter, his body, is subjected to prior scrutiny.

This technique, in effect, borrows a page from the experimental scientist's book. "It is a controlled clinical experiment," Dr. Lawrence Dickey once wrote of the Ecology Unit, "using an individual patient, and has all the validity of a controlled laboratory experiment. Both require control of as many variables as possible."[2]

This may seem like a big job, and indeed it is. First of all, one must control what the patient brings into the hospital. Plastic suitcases, synthetic fabrics, cosmetics, and so forth must all be left behind. Patients can only wear garments made from natural fabrics, such as wool or cotton, and only those which have been washed many times or which were not originally treated with chemicals.

Patients *are* allowed visitors during their stay, which averages three weeks. But the visitors are warned at the door not to enter if they are wearing cosmetics or scent of any kind and not to bring in flowers, candies, or other substances that might make some patients sick or destroy the validity of the test reactions. Staff members, like patients and their visitors, are not allowed to wear any perfumes or scents.

Patients are then fasted on spring water for an average of five days. The purpose of the fast is to completely clear the digestive tract of all food, a process which is often facilitated by the use of milk of magnesia or alkali salts.

In fasting, the patient may experience withdrawal reactions in which his accustomed symptoms get worse for a few days before they get better. The arthritic patient's joints may flare up. The person with a chronic headache problem may suffer a particularly bad attack. The moderately depressed may get a bad attack of the doldrums.

When the worst of the withdrawal reaction is over, however, the patient is tested blindly with several different waters. One of these is the local tap water, and the others are commercially available bottled water (only in glass bottles, never plastic). A new water is tested every three hours, if there has been no adverse reaction to the previous test sample. The patient rates the waters on a scale of zero to ten, without knowing which water he is receiving. He keeps a record of his reactions to the water samples, and the one he tolerates the best will be his compatible water for the remainder of his stay in the hospital. The compatible water is continued on first returning home.

After four or five days, the patient usually feels better; in fact, he may feel healthier than he has in months or years. For example, some patients who have been prostrated by fatigue are able to get up and bustle about. Others who have had pain find that they are virtually pain-free. If the symptoms do not go away, and sometimes they do not, then the fast is prolonged. There is ordinarily no hazard in this, provided that the patient does not have a medical condition which makes fasting dangerous. At all times, of course, the fast is carefully monitored by the medical and nursing staff.

Some fasts have lasted ten days or more. Of course, there are patients whose symptoms are apparently not the result of environmental exposure or for whom even the minimal exposures of the Ecology Unit are disturbing. Such patients may not improve. In the great majority of cases, however, the fast will eventually bring about a cessation of old, disturbing symptoms, and a new sense of well-being, sometimes bordering on the euphoric, will set in. Fasting breaks the addictive cycle of the sick person to the foods and other environmental substances making him ill.

The chemical environment in the Ecology Unit is particularly controlled. Just as there is an attempt to prevent the entry of potentially harmful materials from outside, so too .everything inside the unit is kept as innocuous as can be. This gives the unit a somewhat old-fashioned appearance. The couch in the lounge, for instance, is made of well-worn leather, and the chairs are fashioned from wood and metal, upholstered with cotton or felt, and covered with natural fabrics. All of the bedding is made of simple, untreated cotton, and such things as sponge-rubber pillows or mattresses, draw sheets, upholstered furniture, rug pads, or even tubing made with rubber, are forbidden.

Plastics have also been banished from the Ecology Unit. There are no mattresses with plasticized surfaces, no plastic covers on the pillows, no plastic furniture, shower curtains, drapes, slippers, or handbags.

Initially, there was a problem with the floors. Some of the patients simply did not lose their symptoms, even after a prolonged fast. We finally learned that before the Ecology Unit had taken over this particular space in the hospital, the baseboards had been sprayed with a chemical pesticide. It is virtually impossible to entirely eliminate such sprays. The baseboards and the old floor, therefore, had to go and new tile baseboards and flooring were put down. Since then, far fewer patients have failed to get rid of their symptoms on the fast.

In addition, the Ecology Unit has its own broom closet, and the cleaning personnel use only soap and water. Since there are odors and fumes emanating from other parts of the hospital, it has been necessary to seal off the stairwells, elevator shafts, laundry chutes, and ventilating systems to prevent leakage into the unit. Even the latch holes on the doors were plugged to keep out cigarette smoke. When it is time to paint, the entire floor is evacuated for a week. In addition, large and effective air purifiers are kept running most of the time, despite the fact that the Ecology Unit is located in one of Chicago's least polluted suburbs.

Despite these precautions, chemical contaminants sometimes do get into the unit. Recently, for example, during the shooting of a film, a solvent-based marking pen was opened. Although the pen was not open for more than half a minute, at the next morning's staff meeting one of the nurses reported that several chemically susceptible patients had gotten ill at the time of the shooting. The answer almost certainly lay in this marking pen. When the error was realized, the door and window of the room where the pen was had been foolishly thrown open, blowing the fumes across the hall and into the room opposite. The patients who had gotten ill were in this room. It is because of reactions such as this that great strictness is exercised in controlling chemical pollution of the Ecology Unit.

Food Testing

Once all the variables of the environment have been controlled and the patient is feeling better and has found a compatible water, he is ready to begin his food tests. Generally speaking, the patient breaks his fast with some form of fish, if he has no known allergy to it. It can be either fresh fish or a special form of salmon specifically bottled for the unit in glass.

If this fish is tolerated, the patient is then started on foods which he formerly consumed in some form at least once every three days. During this stage of food testing, the patient is given only organic, chemically less contaminated foods. These are obtained from reliable health food stores. Each meal is made up only of one food, in portions as large as the patient desires. These meals are prepared in stainless steel or glass containers.

The patient is then watched for signs of a reaction. Some foods, even those normally eaten with great frequency, are well tolerated. Others may cause a recurrence of symptoms. The patient is instructed in how to look for and record reactions to these foods. He employs a code, in which reactions are rated either OK (meaning the food is well tolerated), or first, second, third, or fourth degree, indicating the severity and speed of the reactions.

A first degree food produces minor, localized, transient reactions such as a runny nose, itching, mild rash, and so forth. These symptoms are generally of short duration and require no special treatment.

Second degree foods are those which cause a larger number of symptoms, more severe symptoms, or both. These may be either localized or generalized, but are normally not very severe. These symptoms often respond to treatment with alkali salts. Alkali salts are a two-to-one combination of potassium bicarbonate and sodium bicarbonate and are similar to the preparation sold over the counter as aspirin-free "Alka Seltzer Gold." For reasons which are interpreted elsewhere,[3] these salts often have a beneficial, even a dramatic, effect on allergic-type reactions. This relief may last a few hours. Milk of magnesia, which clears the system of offending substances, can also be helpful.

Third degree foods are those which produce a large number of symptoms or more severe reactions. If there is only one symptom but it is very severe or incapacitating, this is also classified as a third degree reaction. For example, any food which puts a patient to sleep is automatically classified as a third degree food, especially if the patient tries to stay awake but cannot.

Reactions in which concentration is altered or in which memory is impaired are designated third degree, because of the importance of these cerebral functions in everyday life. In general, third degree reactions are more severe, generalized, and incapacitating than either of the preceding categories.

A fourth degree reaction is, of course, the worst possible and is either very severe, very rapid in onset, very incapacitating, or all of these. Mania and convulsions are typical plus-four symptoms. Relief of a fourth degree reaction is basically the same as for a third degree, although it might include more vigorous efforts to empty the gastrointestinal tract. Oxygen, which also has a beneficial effect in such circumstances, might also be given.

As has already been indicated in the chapters on "stages and symptoms," contaminated foods can also be used to detect the chemical-susceptibility problem. After the patient has passed his organic food tests, he is then tested on "normal" commercially available foods from the supermarket. The reason for such testing is twofold. First, it takes the average patient about ten days to recover from his formerly almost constant exposure to chemically contaminated foods. Thus, a test of chemically contaminated food early in his visit would not be decisive. Second, it is necessary to be sure that a patient reacting to a chemically contaminated food is reacting to the chemicals and not to the food itself. Organic foods which rated an "OK" in the first testing are thus used as a baseline control to which a patient's reactions to commercially available samples of the same type are compared.

About five percent of the chemically susceptible patients react to their first meal of contaminated ("supermarket") food; about ten percent to their second meal; twenty percent to the third meal; forty percent to the fourth meal; and twenty-five percent to the fifth and sixth meals.

The following commercially available foods are used for testing: raw apples, celery, and lettuce; dietetic canned peaches, cherries, blueberries, and pears; frozen broccoli, cauliflower, brussels sprouts, and spinach; salmon, tuna, and chicken canned in lined tins.

These foods are selected because of their contamination with spray residues and with the golden-colored phenol resins in the linings of the metal cans. In my experience, next to pesticide residue, phenol resins are the most important source of chemical contamination of the food supply.

Chemical Testing

A more direct form of chemical testing is undertaken with certain common petrochemicals found in the environment which are often incriminated in chronic illness. Outside the double swinging doors of the Ecology Unit is a small room in which testing for chemicals is done. Here patients are exposed to the odor of natural gas, similar to what they would experience in a closed kitchen. The patient inhales this air for about a minute and then records changes in pulse (which he is taught to take himself) and the onset of any symptoms.

On various occasions, we test the patient's reaction to the odor of fresh carpeting, which is kept stored in jars, or to torn shreds of carbonless carbon paper, which ordinarily reeks from petrochemicals and is increasingly used in business receipts of all kinds. Patients look for reactions to these chemically impregnated substances and record them the same way they do their reactions to foods.

It has been found that if a patient reacts to one of the common chemicals, he is likely to react to a broad range of petrochemical products. The percentage of patients reacting to chemicals increases year by year as the quality of the environment as a whole declines.

Patients' Participation

The patient is responsible for recording his reactions to the various foods and chemicals according to the instructions which he is given. He is also responsible for other aspects of his own diagnosis and treatment, to an extent unusual in most hospitals.

For example, he is given precise instructions on how to take his own pulse—5 minutes before, and 20, 40, and 60 minutes after the end of each meal. The pulse must be taken for a full minute, and the patient cannot be active or even go to the bathroom immediately before taking it. Any form of physical activity will invalidate the results.

The patient must be disciplined enough not to leave the unit for several weeks nor to eat any substance other than what is ordered for him by the doctor. He also must not smoke at any time while under treatment.

Most of all, the patient must cooperate in *learning*. There is a great deal to learn: new concepts, many of them quite at variance with conventional wisdom on nutrition and health. This is not an easy task for many patients who come to the hospital in a confused or even a bewildered state. They have been sick, often for years, and have usually been through a gamut of unsuccessful medical experiences. Suddenly, they are confronted by concepts and techniques which seem alien to everything that went before.

Unless the patient has some intellectual curiosity, then, it is difficult for him to get the most out of this program. Some patients are so befuddled by their disease that they find it too much of a challenge. Most patients, however, are eager to try something truly different—an alternative approach to their problems.

Complications of Treatment

The complications of this hospital regimen are strikingly few. Occasionally, a patient may decide voluntarily to leave the hospital during the fasting period. This may be the result of an inordinate fear of fasting, the iron grip of some addiction, or an inability to cope with the withdrawal symptoms. There have been a few such instances in which patients left in the midst of acute reactions, following the feeding of a suspected food.

Pregnancy is no problem, however, and pregnant women have been successfully fasted for a few days. Diabetics can also be handled, although in advanced cases the fasts cannot be complete.

In all, patients ranging from young children to elderly people have fasted in our program. Although reactions to foods can be troublesome, it is important to note that no deaths or irreversible complications have ever resulted from this program. Contrast this record to that of conventional medicine, with its emphasis on surgery, radiation, electroshock, and drug therapy. The clinical-ecology approach to chronic illness is logical, effective in many cases, and, above all, safe.

The Placebo Effect

This is all well and good, says the conventional skeptic, but the so-called results of the Ecology Unit, and of clinical ecology, are actually based on suggestion. This is the so-called placebo effect (from the Latin "I will please") in which a totally inert "sugar pill" sometimes has curative properties. In the case of clinical ecology the patient wants to get well to such an extent, we are told, that he accepts the physician's idea that wheat, pork, or some other substance is the source of his illness.

Such arguments are sometimes heard from critics of this new approach, although never yet from a physician who has closely observed our methods nor from a patient who has been treated in the unit. The door of the Ecology

Unit is always open to qualified professionals who wish to investigate our methods first-hand.

The impression of those who have studied the response of patients in our clinic is usually the opposite of those who speculate about the "placebo effect": patients are in fact more likely to respond *negatively* to suggestions that their illness is caused by some common food. Remember, these are not only frequently eaten foods we are talking about, staples in the diet, but more often than not *favorite* foods, which may be eaten in an addictive manner. Patients do not ordinarily encourage doctors to tell them to give up cherished pleasures. Nor do they usually enjoy a new interpretation of their illness which may impinge on their freedom.

The discovery of a food addiction can be unpleasant, for it may mean preparing unaccustomed meals, as well as the chance of social awkwardness. Anyone who thinks patients are easily persuaded to give up their favorite food addictants should try to separate a wheat-a-holic from his bowl of pasta or daily portion of bread.

Similarly, a diagnosis of chemical susceptibility is rarely greeted with enthusiasm by patients. It entails serious changes in lifestyle. Few patients look forward to the opportunity of changing or moving their heating systems, for instance. Their tendency is to *deny* the problem, not to embrace it as one does a placebo. Once a correct diagnosis is made, however, and the patient sees some improvement in his life, he will then often enthusiastically—and rationally—embrace the new regimen.

There is additional evidence that the reactions which patients have to food and chemicals during our testing program are not based on suggestion: blind tests have been performed sufficiently often to prove that such reactions are not dependent on foreknowledge on the part of the patient. Some of the most dramatic of these tests have been recorded on film and shown repeatedly at medical conferences.

Patients have also been given sham feedings through a tube of foods to which they were not allergic or of no food at all, while being told that they were receiving a food to which they were allergic. I have never elicited what appeared to be a psychological reaction from such patients. Invariably, they do *not* react under such circumstances, no matter how they have been primed with suggestion. In one case, discussed at length earlier, I let a beet-sensitive patient glimpse some red juice on a dish after she was given a tube feeding. The dish was then quickly whisked out of her sight and hidden. She failed to react to the feeding, however. When asked if she thought that the feeding had been beets she admitted that she had seen the red juice left in the pan. The juice was actually from a pomegranate and had been deliberately placed in the bowl in an attempt to trigger a psychological reaction.

Other patients have accidentally and unknowingly eaten food to which they were known to be allergic. In these cases, they suffered the same kind of reaction as during a deliberate feeding, although they would have to retrace their steps to discover the cause. Joan Kowan, the student nurse with the headache problem, suffered such an attack after accidentally eating some butter (Chap. 12).

Another case was a physician who suffered from diarrhea whenever he ate milk or milk products. One day he went into a diner and ordered a hamburger and then suffered a reaction. He returned to the diner when he was better, sat himself at the counter, and watched the chef prepare another hamburger. The burger itself contained no milk products, but it was cooked on a griddle still sizzling with butter from the previous order. Even this small amount of a milk product was enough to cause a reaction in him.

Many patients have had similar reactions to coffee, pork, corn, or other foods. Environmental pollutants can unknowingly create symptoms in the same way. Ellen Sanders (Chap. 3) suffered irregular heartbeats (cardiac arrhythmia) after pesticide was drawn into her apartment by an air conditioner. She became deathly ill, but it was not until she was taken to the hospital that it was discovered that these pesticides had been released, in massive quantities, in her vicinity.

It is easy to theorize about psychological effects and placebo reactions. In the Ecology Unit our primary responsibility is in healing the patient, not in performing double blind tests, for which we have neither the facilities nor the funding. It is possible that psychological factors play some unknown role in *all* healing processes. Innumerable facts, however, show that the chronic ailments of patients usually have real causes in the material world, many of which can be unmasked through the methods of clinical ecology.

To summarize, it may be said that the technique of comprehensive environmental control in an isolated hospital unit set up for this task has filled a useful purpose. It is especially helpful for advanced complicated cases in which efforts at outpatient management have failed.

There tends to be a deteriorating continuum in advanced and complicated instances of environmentally related illness which sometimes is difficult to change on the basis of office or outpatient management. This downhill course may often, but not always, be reversed by the application of more detailed observations favored by this approach. It is especially useful in instances where home and work exposures are suspected of maintaining chronic illnesses. Once such chronic manifestations have been reversed, the clinical effects of trial reexposures—either in the hospital or upon returning to home or work conditions—often induce acute convincing test effects.

18

Coping with Food Allergies: The Rotary Diversified Diet

The key to the control of food allergies is the Rotary Diversified Diet. This diet serves three purposes. It is a diagnostic tool, which can unmask hidden food allergies in the course of normal life. It minimizes the development of new allergies, and is thus a preventive measure. And, finally, it helps the patient maintain tolerance to foods he already is able to eat. An individualized program can be worked out for any patient which will help to control the extent and spread of his food allergy. In fact, the Rotary Diversified Diet is more than just a medical maneuver: it is a *life plan* for anyone who wishes to remain well.

This diet was first developed by Dr. Herbert J. Rinkel in 1934. As the name implies, the diet is made up of a highly varied selection of foods. However, these foods are eaten in a definite *rotation*, or order, to prevent the formation of new allergies and to control preexisting ones.

At first, the diet may sound strange to people who have grown used to eating whatever they please, whenever they please. It sets some limits on what you can eat and when you can eat it. On the other hand, it should not be confused with any of the other dietary plans which are currently popular. The Rotary Diversified Diet is not a mass prescription based on sweeping generalization such as "eat less meat," "eat more carbohydrates," or "do not eat sugar." It is an individualized plan, tailor-made for the patient, and for him alone: what works for him may not work for his neighbor.

When allergies to common foods were first discovered, it was natural for doctors to attempt to control them with diets. The type of diets employed in the early part of this century were either mainly diagnostic plans, designed to ferret out a hidden allergy, or treatment plans which left patients with sweeping prohibitions against "nuts," "fish," or "candies." Patients were not told when or how they could reintroduce such foods back into their diets.

Dr. Rinkel devised the Rotary Diversified Diet to fill the void created by these earlier plans. His original purpose in devising the diet was to avoid cumulative reactions. These are food reactions which occur if a person eats the same food over and over again, meal after meal. The constant, monotonous intake of any food promotes the development of a food allergy in a susceptible person. Dr. Rinkel believed that by rotating and diversifying foods, the probability of such problems building up could be minimized.

As he continued to use and evaluate this diet, however, Rinkel soon began to employ it on patients who readily developed *new* food allergies. In mid-1934 he used the diet on a woman patient who suffered from almost constant migraine headaches. She reported that she had not been free of headache for a single day during the previous ten years. Rinkel confirmed the seriousness of her illness by observing her over a period of several months.[1,2]

Rinkel achieved some success in treating her by eliminating first one food to which she was allergic and then another. But then, five to ten days after a suspected food had been eliminated, her symptoms would increase to their previous intensity. Each temporary, partial "cure" was followed by a very disappointing recurrence. What appeared to be happening was that the woman would eliminate one food—wheat, for example—only to develop a new allergy during the next week to her substitute food, oats. The new allergic reaction would bring back the original headache.

To prevent this from happening, Rinkel suggested she try something new. Specifically, he told her to *diversify* her diet, so that she ate many foods. He also instructed her to *rotate* her foods, that is, to repeat them only at specified intervals. If she ate corn at one meal she would have to, in effect, give her body a rest and not eat corn in any form for several more days. (Originally the interval ranged from one to three days: today it is generally longer.)

Within a few years, Rinkel was joined by a small but dedicated circle of allergists also employing the new technique. I myself began using the diet for my patients in the early 1940s. I have put thousands of people on this diet, and have seen the beneficial results it brings in the great majority of cases.

In devising a rotary diet for patients, I follow certain basic rules. Patients are instructed in these rules and given advice on how to follow them when they return home.

Rule 1: Eat whole, unadulterated foods. Our ancestors generally ate their food in a simple form, without complicated mixtures, sauces, condiments, and the like. A diet such as this is cheaper, more readily available, easier to prepare, and more digestible than fancier fare.

Today, most of us have the ability to eat both simply *and* with variety. Culinary refinement, while pleasing to the palate, can sometimes be harmful to health, if it is pursued on a regular basis by susceptible individuals. The overrefinement of foods and their packaging for convenience or longer shelf life have led to abuses. Many people do not know what a diet of plain, simple foods taste like or how good it can be. If a person tolerates beef, he can and should enjoy a steak, a hamburger, or a piece of boiled beef instead of, say, a meatball sandwich. If he eats steak, he has consumed one food—beef. He can then have another food, or several other foods, for his next meal. But the meatballs may contain beef, soy, pork, onion, oil, butter, milk, egg, black pepper, and wheat flour used as a "meat-stretcher." The bread will contain more wheat, rye, corn oil, yeast, sugar of some sort, caramel, lactic-acid cultures, and assorted chemicals. If the sandwich is topped with catsup, it will contain tomatoes, vinegar (grain, cider, or wine), corn sweetener, onion powder, spices, and flavorings. Mayonnaise will add more eggs and vinegar, as well as soybean oil and sugar (beet or cane).

Thus, what most people think of as a fairly simple meal—a meatball sandwich such as is available in many restaurants or "take-out" places—actually may contain more than two dozen different foods, including some of the most common allergy-causing substances—wheat, corn, beef, beet, milk, cane, yeast, soy, or eggs. Most likely it will also contain an assortment of chemicals as well.

If you are allergic to any one of these common items (and almost all food allergy patients are), you will not be able to discover this fact by sticking to the average American diet. The reason is that you will eat these common foods over and over again, every day, almost without letup. The symptoms caused by one or more of these foods may fluctuate, but they will never really be absent for long, because their cause is not absent for long. If you find that an average meal gives you reaction, it will be virtually impossible to track down the cause of that reaction when you are eating two dozen different foods at a sitting.

Rule 2: Diversify your diet. In addition to eating whole, simple foods, the patient must learn to diversify his diet. The modern marketplace offers us a wide variety of different foods from various climates and cultures. We should make use of this diversity. Yet most people eat the same few foods over and over again, sometimes quite literally ad nauseam. Wheat, milk, beef, corn, beet or cane sugars, and eggs, in their many varieties and disguises, represent the monotonous basis of the American diet. Some people even brag of being "meat and potato men," who must have these two foods in order to feel satisfied (an almost certain sign of food addiction).

Patients can learn to diversify their food choices. The world is filled with an enticing variety of foods which they can exploit for both enjoyment and good health. For example, few people enjoy (or have even tasted) all of the foods in a well-stocked fruit and vegetable market. They become stuck on certain often-repeated favorites, such as carrots, celery, and lettuce, and bypass what is unfamiliar. Turnips and parsnips are rarely eaten as vegetables in their own right, although they make a delicious dish. Some people have never tasted artichokes, avocados, mangos, or papayas. Each of these can form the basis of a satisfying meal.

Some foods are only eaten on special occasions or in special combinations. Cranberries are highly popular at Thanksgiving, but are rarely eaten at any other time of the year; yet they can usually be incorporated into the diet with little trouble, and in many markets they can be purchased fresh throughout the fall season.

The foods of other countries offer interesting possibilities. Many markets now carry bean sprouts (mung or alfalfa) and (soy) bean curd. Bean sprouts can be readily grown in a jar in the kitchen if they are not available in the store. Health food stores usually stock a wide variety of Japanese foods. The larger cities have stores, listed in the Yellow Pages, which sell specialty foods of other nationalities. There is much to be gained by learning to enjoy the cuisine of cultures other than one's own.

In fact, the Rotary Diversified Diet is in some ways less limited, and more enjoyable, than the supposedly unrestricted but monotonous American diet. It calls on you to eat in a controlled, rational way, but within that plan it offers great latitude for innovation and experimentation with food.

Rule 3: Rotate your diet. Patients are told that they can develop an allergy to any food if they eat it day in and day out and are susceptible to it. This is as true of the more exotic foods as it is of beef, potatoes, or eggs. A colleague of mine once attempted to practice clinical ecology in Taiwan. He soon discovered that the Chinese people of that island had widespread allergies to the foods eaten there, especially soy and rice, but also including others, some of which are rare by American standards.

The whole point of this diet is to let the body recover from the effects of a food before eating it again. In general, it takes up to three days for a meal to pass through the human digestive system. To be safe, we allow four days between ingestions of a particular food.

In general, patients are instructed to have only three meals per day. They can eat as much as they wish, although they are encouraged to eat portions of normal size. (The diet is also an excellent way to lose weight.)

If he follows a four-day rotation, the patient can eat a particular food on Monday and then eat it again on Friday. Thus, if he has wheat on Monday, he will have to count four days following Monday before he can have wheat again. Bear in mind that this means wheat *in any form:* bread, spaghetti, lasagna, cream of wheat, even the breading on a pork chop. It is important to add that, for the purposes of this diet, wheat is identical to rye, barley, malt, and millet. Of course, if the patient continues to eat the average American diet, he could not manage that, since there is wheat (or a related grain) in almost every typical meal. But on the Rotary Diversified Diet, it is not difficult to avoid unknown or unsuspected ingredients in foods.

While four days is what we might call the "legal limit" on food repetition, many patients go on a seven-day cycle. This allows them to eat the same basic diet each week. The diet can be posted on the refrigerator and is easy to follow. All the patient needs to begin a seven-day food cycle are twenty-one foods to which he is not allergic.

Rule 4: Rotate food families. Foods, whether animal or vegetable, come in families. Some of these are fairly obvious: cabbage, kale, broccoli, and cauliflower, for example, all taste somewhat similar and are clearly related. You probably would not guess, however, that they are in the mustard family, which also includes horseradish and watercress. Similarly, you would not automatically know that cashews, pistachios, and mangoes are in the same group or that beef and lamb are in the same family but that deer and elk are in a separate group.

Food families are important in devising a Rotary Diversified Diet. A listing of common foods, grouped by their families, is given in Appendix A, to convey some idea of the relations between various foods.

The reason food families are important is that patients can cross-react to the "relatives" of food to which they are allergic. Thus, if you are allergic to beef you must suspect goat (not to mention veal and milk, both of which are seen as similar to beef by the body—veal being young beef, and milk a product of the female of the species). People who are allergic to potato must suspect other members of its family, including tomato, green pepper, red pepper, chili, eggplant, and tobacco. (Tobacco, however, should be shunned by everybody.)

Another reason why it is important to be aware of food families is to prevent the formation of allergies by a steady consumption of foods which are members of the same family. If you eat tomato on Monday, eggplant on Tuesday, potato on Wednesday, green pepper on Thursday, and tomato again on Friday, you are not really rotating foods—you are eating from the same food family every day, and this could develop into an addiction to one or all of these items.

Thus, the ingestion of foods which are members of the same family must be spaced, but not quite as strictly as foods themselves. The rule is that the patient must *rotate food-family members every two days.* Using the above example, it might be perfectly all right to have tomato on Monday, eggplant on Wednesday, and tomato again on Friday, provided that no other members of this family were eaten in between.

If a patient has a known allergy to a particular food, he must also avoid the other members of that food family, at least for a while. Thus, sensitivity to beef brings with it a ban on beef, beef by-products such as gelatin, margarine, and suet, milk products, veal, buffalo, goat, lamb, or mutton.

Rule 5: Eat only foods to which you are not allergic, at first. Patients who are emerging from the Ecology Unit (Chap. 17) are given a summary of their food-test reactions. They therefore know which of the most common foods cause reactions and which do not.

Upon going home, one of their goals is to test other foods which were not evaluated in their weeks in the hospital. If a new food causes no reactions, then it can be added to the Rotary Diversified Diet to give greater variety to the meal plan.

On the other hand, the diet serves as a perpetual diagnostic screen, helping patients to avoid unsuspected sources of mental and physical complaints. It can readily detect the first signs of an adverse reaction to any food, since that food is not in one's system at the time it is eaten.

Basically, there are two kinds of food allergies—fixed and nonfixed, or temporary. A fixed allergy is one with which you are probably born, which does not go away with time. These are relatively less common. More frequently, patients can regain tolerance to troublesome foods after a period of some months of avoidance. The greater the reaction to a food, the longer it takes, in general, to reestablish tolerance. The process usually takes from two to eight months, after which the food can usually be eaten again, if used in rotation. Since the incriminated food is often a favorite and is craved in an addictive manner, the hope of regaining tolerance to it offers some consolation to the patient suffering its temporary loss. Until and unless such tolerance is regained, however, the patient cannot safely use an allergenic food. Moreover, it must not be abused by cumulative intake when it is returned. Re-sensitization occurs very readily and very subtly.[2]

One exception to this rule is the so-called universal reactor. As mentioned earlier, such a person is allergic to *all* or most foods, and will get sick no matter what he eats, although he feels tolerably well on a fast. Naturally, he cannot avoid all foods to which he is allergic or he will starve. In this case, we do the next best thing. He is instructed to eat only those foods to which he has lesser reactions.

In addition, other procedures can be employed to benefit such patients. Some clinical ecologists employ "neutralizing doses" in the treatment of this condition. As was previously explained, a "neutralizing dose" is an infinitesimally small amount of the offending substance. If this dose, placed under the tongue, is at just the right dilution, it will have the effect of turning off a reaction. The same substance in a larger dose will, of course, cause a renewal of symptoms.

This seems contradictory, but the effectiveness of the neutralizing dose is attested to by many clinical ecologists (see Chap. 16).

With the exception of universal reactors, all patients are instructed to keep away from the foods which cause their reactions until these can safely be reworked into the diet.

With these five rules in mind, patients are instructed in how to construct a Rotary Diversified Diet to fit their needs. The diet is an essential part of their treatment. Construction of the diet is essential for such patients, and I employ several well-trained registered nurses whose job it is to instruct patients on the construction of the plan.

It has been explained that four days is a sufficient interval between feedings of any particular food, and that a patient can eat any food to which he is not allergic, provided that he sticks by the rules of rotation. Thus, if a patient wishes, he could have quite a few foods at a meal and then repeat that same meal four days later, *provided* he did not have any of those foods in the intervening time.

For the sake of simplicity, however, let us make the time interval in the following sample diet seven days. Also, for the sake of this presentation, let us assume that the patient eats only one food per meal. This is, of course, not necessary. If he has the tolerance, he can eat a number of foods at each meal.

Following the above-mentioned rules, the patient with at least twenty-one tolerated foods can construct a Rotary Diversified Diet for himself. Here is one such sample diet:

	Sunday	Monday	Tuesday	Wednesday	Thursday	Friday	Saturday
Breakfast	Fresh or frozen melon	Poached eggs	Natural applesauce (no sugar)	Hot oatmeal	Orange slices, plus orange juice	Fresh grapes, plus grape juice	Grapefruit, plus grapefruit juice
Lunch	Steamed broccoli	Cracked wheat porridge	Cooked lima beans	Steamed zucchini (squash) slices	Black-eyed peas	Boiled brown rice	Baked flounder
Dinner	Boiled shrimp	Broiled steak	Pork chops	Chicken	Salmon steaks	Lamb chops	Fresh leg of turkey

You will notice that no food is repeated during the week. Also, no two members of a food family are eaten two days in succession. For example, eggs and chicken are in the same family, but eggs are eaten on Monday and chicken on Wednesday. Squash and melon are related, but they too are separated by a day, as are wheat and oatmeal.

Remember, also, that "apples" means apple *in any form*. At this meal, the patient can have whole apples, apple juice, applesauce, and so forth, provided that the dish to be consumed contains *nothing else*. If anything else is added, it must be counted as a separate food. In other words, if the person sprinkles cinnamon on top of the applesauce, this counts as an item in the Rotary Diversified Diet, and it must be eaten in accordance with the rules. This would mean, for example, that the patient could not have cinnamon again for four days, or members of the cinnamon family (avocado, bay leaf, sassafras) for two days. If sugar is added to the applesauce, this eliminates that type of sugar for four days. One of the dangers of eating commercially prepared foods is that labels are not required to state *what kind* of sugar has been added to food. It is therefore best to avoid foods to which sugars have been added.

It must be emphasized that cane, beet, and corn sugar are specific foods,[3] although cane and beet sugar are chemically indistinguishable, both being called sucrose. In contrast to these double sugars, corn sugar is a molecule one-half their size, most commonly called dextrose, glucose, corn sweetener, or fructose (although fructose for intravenous purposes is usually made from sucrose).

It is a good idea, for the sake of variety, to eat a food in a number of different forms at any one meal. In addition, if the patient cooks his meat in a tolerated water he can then drink the resulting juice hot as a delicious soup. Salt can be added to taste, since salt is one food to which people rarely develop allergies. However, salt should not be used excessively by anyone.

In the above basic diet, I have chosen fairly "normal" foods for each time of the day. For example, most people already eat such things as eggs, melons, and oranges for breakfast. Americans are also accustomed to eating their heavier, meat dishes in the evening. Remember, however, that this is purely conventional. There is no physiological reason to do this and, in fact, in different cultures people have different ideas about what constitutes an acceptable breakfast food, or when people should eat their biggest meal.

Patients are therefore urged to break with food stereotypes when preparing meals. For example, one can eat a piece of plain poached fish, such as flounder or cod, for breakfast. At other breakfasts, one can have meat or vegetables. Flexibility in this regard helps the patient succeed in following the plan.

The diet given above assumes that the patient is not allergic to any of the listed foods. But what if he is allergic to some of them, as is likely, since this chart contains some of the most common allergy-causing foods? In that case, the patient must substitute other foods of known safety, or foods which he is about to test for compatibility. Let us say, for example, that the patient is allergic to all grains and to pork. In that case, his Rotary Diversified Diet might look like this:

	Sunday	Monday	Tuesday	Wednesday	Thursday	Friday	Saturday
Breakfast	Fresh or frozen melon	Poached eggs	Natural applesauce (no sugar)	Pineapple (instead of oatmeal)	Orange slices, plus orange juice	Fresh grapes, plus grape juice	Grapefruit, plus grape-fruit juice
Lunch	Steamed broccoli	Dates (instead of wheat)	Cooked lima beans	Steamed zucchini (squash) slices	Black-eyed peas	Bananas (instead of rice)	Baked flounder
Dinner	Boiled shrimp	Broiled steak	Baked yams (instead of pork)	Chicken	Salmon steaks	Lamb chops	Fresh leg of turkey

Is such a diet balanced? In my opinion, it is. There is an adequate amount of carbohydrate, calories, protein, and other food constituents over the course of a week to maintain health. Does the patient get enough vitamins and minerals on such a diet? In my experience, the consumption of whole (and especially organic) foods, served fresh, will provide better nutrition than the average American diet, even when the latter is supplemented with vitamin pills. In general, I do not recommend vitamin supplements to patients on this diet.

Although some vitamins are made from foods, the majority are manufactured synthetically. The Food and Drug Administration, which regulates this area, does not distinguish between so-called natural and synthetic vitamins, since both have the same structural chemical formulas. If the vitamin is made from sprouted wheat (as are some of the B-vitamin supplements), you may be creating or perpetuating a susceptibility to cereal grain. This is a fact which is overlooked by many vitamin proponents.

I am not against vitamins—far from it. But I believe it is always preferable to obtain vitamins from their natural source, in whole foods, rather than through a supplement, which may contain traces of various chemicals or foods, including additives (cornstarch, milk lactose, and so forth) that can aggravate allergic problems.

The Rotary Diversified Diet represents a profound step forward in man's understanding of how to eat. For millennia, man ate what came to hand, and did well—well enough to survive, at least. In the last few thousand years, however, civilization has altered man's eating patterns and in many ways disrupted our natural balance with the environment. It has taken science to show us how to eat properly under these new conditions. The first big breakthrough was analytical nutrition. This is the nutrition taught in most schools and preached in newspapers, on television, and in numerous books and articles. According to this concept, all food can be reduced to certain neatly defined constituents in pigeon-holed categories—proteins, carbohydrates, vitamins, and the like. An adequate diet, according to this school of thought, is one which provides a given *quantity* of these various nutrients every twenty-four hours. Ross Hume Hall calls this "adding machine" dietetics.

This theory fails to take into account the individual nature of foods and, in particular, the individual nature of each human being. The reaction between the unique individual and his environment is what really matters, especially to a sick person and his physician. This orientation is best referred to as biologic dietetics or nutrition.[4]

Clinical ecology shows us how to restore the balance between man and his environment under the conditions of advanced civilization. It recognizes the unique aspects of both sides of this interaction, including the still unexplored way in which the human body can "recognize" a particular food, even in its most disguised forms.

The Rotary Diversified Diet is the outcome of this new perspective. It is a breakthrough in medicine at least as important as the discovery of "adding-machine" nutrition. It is at once our best means of diagnosis, treatment, and prevention of chronic food reactions.

19

The Chemical Questionnaire

As part of their medical history, all patients are asked to fill out the following Chemical Questionnaire. The answers to these questions serve as a guide to future therapy and prevention. A strongly positive questionnaire, for example, might indicate that the patient should be hospitalized for further diagnosis in the Ecology Unit. The number of positive responses is also used to determine which dilution of synthetic ethyl alcohol should be given in the provocative test (see Chap. 16).

Ideally, the Chemical Questionnaire should be given before the patient knows too much about the overall chemical-susceptibility problem. At least, this has traditionally been the goal. As the problem of chemical susceptibility gains greater prominence, this becomes less possible. You might try filling out this questionnaire yourself, or trying it on a friend or relative who is thought to have this problem. Bear in mind, however, that positive answers on the questionnaire itself only indicate that a problem may exist. They are a good signal to seek further professional help, and to institute some of the preventive techniques outlined in Chapter 20.

This section of the questionnaire can provide some very revealing information, although at first sight the questions appear commonplace. If there is a passageway between the house and the garage, for instance, this could provide an inlet for noxious automobile fumes into the dwelling space.

The questions about the heating system are among the most important in the entire questionnaire. Very often the bulk of a person's problem can be traced to a faulty heating system, with its accompanying hydrocarbon pollution. An oil-impregnated air conditioner filter can be the source of unsuspected room pollution.

If the kitchen has a gas range or a gas refrigerator and does not have an

Human Ecology and Susceptibility to the Chemical Environment Questionnaire

CHEMICAL ADDITIVES AND CONTAMINANTS OF AIR, FOOD, WATER, DRUGS, AND COSMETICS

Date _____ Name _____   Home Address _____

CIRCLE or FILL IN the following: Sex _____ Age _____

Education		*Marital Status*	*Occupation* _____
Highest school year:		Single	*Work Region* *Work Address*
1 2 3 4 5 6 7 8	1 2 3 4	Married	City Distance from work _____
Elementary	High	Widowed	Suburban *Travel by:*
1 2 3 4	1 2 3 4	Separated	Small town Car Train Other _____
College	Graduate	Divorced	Rural Bus Walking _____

Home

Type	*If multiple dwelling*	*Region*	*Garage*
Single House	What floor? _____	City residential	In separate unattached
Double House	How long have you	City industrial	building
Apartment	lived there? _____	Suburban	With inside passageway
Hotel	_____	Small town	between house & garage
Trailer		Rural	In basement of house

Heating & Ventilation of Home

Type	*Fuel*	*Furnace*	*Air Conditioning*	*Kitchen Exhaust*
Electric, heat pump	Electric	*Location*	Window units	*Fan*
Electric, radiant	Gas	Basement	Central system	Yes
Hot water or steam	Oil	Main floor	Filters—Oiled	No
Warm air	Coal	Utility room	Unoiled	*Kitchen Door*
Space heaters	Wood	Open	Electrostatic	Usually left open
Fireplaces	Other ____	Closed	Activated carbon	Usually closed

Utilities

Range	*Refrigerator*		*Deep Freeze*	*Clothes dryer*	*Water Heater*
Electric	*Type*	*Food Storage*	Electric	Electric	Electric
Gas	Electric	In Glass	Gas	Gas	Gas
Oil	Gas	In enamel ware	Age ____	Age ____	Part of furnace
Age ____	Age ____	In plastic			Age ____

Furnishings and Household Maintenance

Upholstery		*Mattresses*	*Pillows*	*Rugs*	*Rug Pads*
Coverings	*Padding*	Cotton	Feather	Wool	Plastic
Cotton Silk	Cotton	Rubber	Rubber	Cotton	Rubber
Linen Wool	Hair	Plastic covered	Kapok	Synthetic	Hair
Synthetic fabrics	Rubber	Other _____	Dacron	Natural fiber	
Plastic	Other ____		Plastic covered	Rubber or	
				Plastic backed	

Curtains	*Cleansers*	*Deodorants &*	*Laundry*		*Furniture*
Cotton silk	Soap	*Disinfectants*	Soap	Plastic starch	*Polish*
Wool linen	Detergents	Air wick	Bleaches	Cornstarch	Yes No
Plastic	Scouring pwd.	Lysol	Ammonia	*Dryer*	*Floor Wax*
Synthetic	with bleach	Pine-Sol	Detergents	Electric	Yes No
material	Ammonia	Others _____		Gas	

Miscellaneous				
Insect Control	*Drinking Water*	*Sense of Smell*	*Ability to Detect*	*When Wind is*
Sprays	Spring or well	Very acute	*Leaking Gas*	*Blowing from*
Moth Balls	Softened	Normal	Acute	*Industrial Areas*
Moth Crystals	Chlorinated	Poor	Normal or average	Are your symptoms
Exterminators	Fluoridated	Absent	Poor or absent	Increased?
				Unchanged?

exhaust fan, this could be another likely source of chemical pollution. If the kitchen door is kept open, trace amounts of natural gas or cooking odors can circulate throughout the entire house, affecting the health of all those in the apartment or dwelling.

The nature of home furnishings and household maintenance equipment also has a very important influence on health, as has been stressed in preceding chapters. If a patient tends to use natural fibers and fabrics, such as cotton, silk, linen, and wool, there is less likelihood of accentuating the chemical-susceptibility problem than if he uses synthetics and plastics.

An all foam rubber bed and foam rubber pillow, or one made from Kapok, Dacron, or plastic-covered materials, can be a source of significant trouble. (Remember, each of us spends approximately one-third of his life in close proximity to bedding.)

The presence of synthetic rugs and carpets and odorous plastic or foam-rubber rug pads has been correlated with numerous ecological problems in the past, and a positive answer here provides a clue.

Many cleansers and detergents are unsuspected sources of problems, as are furniture polishes and floor waxes.

The methods used for insect control in a patient's home come under intense scrutiny. Are there moth balls and crystals in the closet? Does he use an insect spray or keep any under the kitchen sink? Does he have roach or ant traps scattered around the house? Is the house itself resting on a foundation treated with such pesticides as Aldrin and Dieldrin? Does he have a contract with an exterminator who regularly sprays behind the refrigerator, the cabinets, and around the baseboards? This section of the questionnaire is meant to reveal such trouble spots.

The domestic water supply is very important, and in fact some people cannot even bathe or wash their faces with chlorinated water, much less drink it.

The questions about smell rank among the most important in the entire questionnaire and answers to them are the most indicative of a potential chemical problem. People with either a very acute sense of smell or a *poor or absent* sense of smell are likely to be highly susceptible to chemicals. The typical allergy patient usually starts with a hyperacute sense of smell. This may eventually become overwhelmed, however, by exposure to chemical fumes and smells, so that eventually the patient has *no* sense of smell. There is no contradiction here: rather, the two extremes are part of a process, a syndrome, and it is the doctor's role to explain how that syndrome developed over a period of time. Of the various questions concerning the sense of smell, the ability to detect leaking gas is one of the most important. Again, if the patient is the kind of person who is constantly sniffing the air and complaining that he smells gas when no one else can, even when gas-company meters show no leak, then there is a good chance that he is chemically susceptible. In fact, it is likely that it is precisely this natural gas which is causing some (or all) of his symptoms. If, on the other hand, he cannot smell gas when others can, or has *lost* his ability to smell it, this may also be a sign of a chemical-susceptibility problem, at a different stage.

Unpleasant smells themselves may cause allergic-type reactions. According to Iris Bell, Ph.D. (also M.D.), a researcher in this field, odors

> can directly influence the function of a wide variety of central nervous system reactions. It might be speculated that specific odors could excessively stimulate or depress certain [brain] circuits to produce the manic-depressive swings of mood seen in some ecologic patients.[1]

In answering the following questions, it is helpful if you also indicate in the right margin the major type of symptoms which you associate with a given exposure. Such replies might indicate running nose, coughing, wheezing, nausea, itching, headache, brain-fag, depression, etc.

What Is Your Reaction to the Following?

	Check One: Like	Neu-tral	Dis-like	Made sick from
Coal, Oil, Gas, & Combustion Products				
1. Massive outdoor exposures to coal smoke	____	____	____	____
2. Smoke in steam railroad stations, train sheds, and yards	____	____	____	____
3. Smoke from coal burning stoves, furnaces, or fireplaces	____	____	____	____
4. Odors of natural gas fields	____	____	____	____
5. Odors of escaping utility gas	____	____	____	____
6. Odors of burning utility gas	____	____	____	____
7. Odors of gasoline	____	____	____	____
8. Garage fumes and odors	____	____	____	____
9. Automotive or motor boat exhausts	____	____	____	____
10. Odor of naphtha, cleaning fluids, or lighter fluids	____	____	____	____

Check One:	Like	Neu- tral	Dis- like	Made sick from

11. Odor of recently cleaned clothing, up-
holstery, or rugs.................................. _____ _____ _____ _____
12. Odor of naphtha-containing soaps............... _____ _____ _____ _____
13. Odor of nail polish or nail polish re-
mover.. _____ _____ _____ _____
14. Odor of brass, metal, or shoe polishes.......... _____ _____ _____ _____
15. Odor of fresh newspapers....................... _____ _____ _____ _____
16. Odor of kerosene .... _____ _____ _____ _____
17. Odor of kerosene or fuel-oil burning
lamps or stoves................................ _____ _____ _____ _____
18. Odor of kerosene or fuel-oil burning
space heaters or furnaces....................... _____ _____ _____ _____
19. Diesel engine fumes from trains, busses,
trucks, or boats .... _____ ● _____ _____
20. Lubricating greases or crude oil .... _____ _____ _____ _____
21. Fumes from automobiles burning an ex-
cessive amount of oil........................... _____ _____ _____ _____
22. Fumes from burning greasy rags .... _____ _____ _____ _____
23. Odors of smudge pots as road markers
or frost inhibitors .... _____ _____ _____

The above set of questions refers to the role of petrochemical fumes and by-products as causes of illness. Here the questionnaire seeks information not about whether the patient can detect the odors, but about how he reacts to them. So-called subjective reactions of like and dislike are often indicative of processes taking place within the body.

Again, the patient may have seemingly contradictory reactions to various substances. Often, the patient will start out *liking* the very substance which is making him ill. Eventually, he may develop a profound dislike for that substance, which may strike the uninformed observer as "irrational" or "paranoid."

Some people, for instance, crave the smell (and the effects) of raw gasoline, even making a point to get out of the car and stand by the pumps while their tank is being filled. In time, however, they may find they become nauseated or develop a headache simply by entering a service station.

What Is Your Reaction to the Following?

Check One:	Like	Neu- tral	Dis- like	Made sick from

**Mineral Oil, Vaseline, Waxes, &
Combustion Products**
1. Mineral oil as contained in hand lotions
and medications .... _____ _____ _____ _____
2. Mineral oil as a laxative .... _____ _____ _____ _____

Check One:	Like	Neu- tral	Dis- like	Made sick from
3. Cold cream or face or foundation cream	____	____	____	____
4. Vaseline, petroleum jelly, or petrolatum- containing ointments	____	____	____	____
5. Odors of floor, furniture, or bowling alley wax.....................................	____	____	____	____
6. Odors of glass wax or similar glass cleaners	____	____	____	____
7. Fumes from burning wax candles	____	____	____	____
8. Odors from dry garbage incinerators	____	____	____	____

Many people do not realize that mineral oil is derived from petroleum, just as gasoline and motor oil are. Mineral oil, either swallowed as a laxative or applied to the skin, can be the source of allergic-type reactions. (It can also cause cancer. Workers in the cotton industry once contracted scrotal cancer at over one hundred times the average rate when mineral oils were cast as a fine spray onto their groins and forearms. When the type of oil was changed, this occupational hazard virtually disappeared.[2])

Many cold creams, face creams, and foundation creams, as well as various home and commercial waxes also contain petroleum products, and should be carefully avoided by those susceptible to such products. Natural substitutes are available in most cases.

What Is Your Reaction to the Following?

Check One:	Like	Neu- tral	Dis- like	Made sick from
Asphalts, Tars, Resins, & Dyes				
1. Fumes from tarring roofs and roads	____	____	____	____
2. Asphalt pavements in hot weather	____	____	____	____
3. Tar-containing soaps, shampoos, and oint- ments..	____	____	____	____
4. Odors of inks, carbon paper, typewriter ribbons, and stencils	____	____	____	____
5. Dyes in clothing and shoes	____	____	____	____
6. Dyes in cosmetics (lipstick, mascara, rouge, powder, other)	____	____	____	____

Tar can be a significant problem for motorists. Many chemically susceptible patients have become acutely ill when they are driving over a stretch of freshly tarred road or have been caught behind a tar truck in traffic. In the summertime, asphalt pavements may have a tendency to soften or even melt and can cause problems for the unwary.

People with such susceptibilities must definitely avoid tar-containing soaps, shampoos, and ointments, which add little in the way of cleaning capacity and can cause serious health problems.

The odors of inks, carbon paper, typewriter ribbons, and stencils constitute an obvious danger to secretaries and others working in offices. Dr. Guy O. Pfeiffer has made a study of environmental hazards in the typical office. The copy machine, he reports, uses inks, dyes, and chemicals which may give off a chemical gas. The printed page which comes out of the machine has a characteristic odor. The material from which the paper is made, as well as the ink, when fresh, will "gas out" for a while.

In addition, he notes the presence of spray cans for various purposes in the average office, "the can of a thousand labels, a thousand ingredients, and potentially a thousand different problems to the chemically sensitive individual."[3]

Newspapers, carpeting, synthetically covered upholstery, tobacco smoke, potted plants, insecticides, sanitizers, and other sources of chemical fumes must all be considered in making a diagnosis of chemical susceptibility. The above questions provide the physician with a clue and a starting point for further investigation.

Dyes in cosmetics, such as lipstick, mascara, and rouge, are often implicated in patients' problems, and even "hypoallergenic" products can cause reactions.

What Is Your Reaction to the Following?

Check one:	Like	Neu-tral	Dis-like	Made Sick from
Disinfectants, Deodorants, & Detergents				
1. Odor of public or household disinfectants and deodorants	____	____	____	____
2. Odor of phenol (carbolic acid) or Lysol	____	____	____	____
3. Phenol-containing lotions or ointments	____	____	____	____
4. Injectable materials containing phenol as a preservative	____	____	____	____
5. Fumes from burning creosote-treated wood (railroad ties)	____	____	____	____
6. Household detergents	____	____	____	____

Phenol, or carbolic acid, is of particular concern to physicians, and especially clinical ecologists. This is because most of the extracts used in the provocative/neutralizing tests are preserved with phenol. Many biological drugs, in addition, must by law be preserved with phenol. If a patient is susceptible to phenol, it may be necessary to prepare special extracts without this preservative. As previously mentioned, in addition to its other uses, phenol is used in the lining of food cans. A patient who indicates a like or dislike for phenol as a disinfectant may also react to the ever more common presence of phenol as a food contaminant.

What Is Your Reaction to the Following?

	Check One: Like	Neu- tral	Dis- like	Made sick from
Rubber				
1. Odor of rubber or contact with rubber— gloves, elastic in clothing, girdles, brassieres, garters, etc.	___	___	___	___
2. Odor of sponge-rubber bedding, rug pads, typewriter pads	___	___	___	___
3. Odor of rubber-based paint	___	___	___	___
4. Odor of rubber tires, automotive acces- sories, etc.	___	___	___	___
5. Odor of rubber-backed rugs and carpets	___	___	___	___
6. Fumes of burning rubber	___	___	___	___

Rubber is another common source of problems. As most people know, today's rubber is only rarely the natural, plant-derived latex. In the vast majority of cases, it is a synthetic substance, derived from various chemicals and petroleum by-products.

What Is Your Reaction to the Following?

	Check One: Like	Neu- tral	Dis- like	Made sick from
Plastics, Synthetic Textiles, Finishes, & Adhesives				
1. Odor of or contact with plastic upholstery, tablecloths, book covers, pillow covers, shoe bags, handbags	___	___	___	___
2. Odor of plastic folding doors or interiors of automobiles	___	___	___	___
3. Odor of or contact with plastic spectacle frames, dentures	___	___	___	___
4. Odor of plastic products in department or specialty stores	___	___	___	___
5. Nylon hose and other nylon wearing apparel	___	___	___	___
6. Dacron or Orlon clothing or upholstery	___	___	___	___
7. Rayon or cellulose-acetate clothing or upholstery	___	___	___	___
8. Odor of or contact with adhesive tape	___	___	___	___
9. Odor of plastic cements	___	___	___	___

Plastics, of course, constitute one of the most common sources of chemical exposure. An increasing number of commercial products are made from plastics, many of which are described elsewhere in this book. These questions are designed to show the patient's reaction to some of the most obvious sources of plastic exposure. Reactions to plastic can be varied and extreme.

What Is Your Reaction to the Following?

	Check One: Like	Neu-tral	Dis-like	Made sick from
Alcohols, Glycols, Aldehydes, Ketones, Esters, Terpines, & Derived Substances				
1. Odor of rubbing alcohol	____	____	____	____
2. Alcohols or glycols as contained in medications	____	____	____	____
3. Odor of varnish, lacquer, or shellac	____	____	____	____
4. Odor of drying paint	____	____	____	____
5. Odor of after-shave hair tonics or hair oils.......................................	____	____	____	____
6. Odor of window cleaning fluids..................	____	____	____	____
7. Odor of paint or varnish thinned with mineral solvents..................................	____	____	____	____
8. Odor of banana oil (amyl alcohol)	____	____	____	____
9. Odor of scented soap and shampoo..............	____	____	____	____
10. Odor of perfumes and colognes..................	____	____	____	____
11. Odor of Spray Net® and other hair dressings	____	____	____	____
12. Fumes from burning incense....................	____	____	____	____

Most perfumes, colognes, and scented commercial products are primarily mixes of synthetically derived materials. It is rare today to find an entirely biological perfume. Although some brands of perfume are more troublesome to the chemically susceptible person than others, rarely are any of them tolerated by the highly susceptible.

A hand lotion or any ointment may be troublesome for the chemically susceptible patient on several scores—because of the artificial colors (dyes), scents, preservatives, emulsifiers as well as both the active and inactive materials in the formula.

Reactions to paints and varnishes are largely based on the volatility of solvents incorporated in their manufacture. However, even a biological solvent such as turpentine may still be troublesome; this is part of the pine problem.

What Is Your Reaction to the Following?

	Check One: Like	Neu-Tral	Dis-like	Made sick from
Miscellaneous				
1. Air conditioning	____	____	____	____
2. Ammonia fumes................................	____	____	____	____
3. Odor of moth balls	____	____	____	____
4. Odor of insect-repellant candles	____	____	____	____
5. Odor of termite extermination treatment.................................	____	____	____	____

	Check One:		Neu-	Dis-	Made sick
		Like	tral	like	from
6. Odor of DDT-containing insecticide sprays		____	____	____	____
7. Odor of Chlordane, Lindane, Parathione, Dieldrin, and other insecticide sprays		____	____	____	____
8. Odor of weed killers (herbicides)		____	____	____	____
9. Odor of the fruit and vegetable sections of supermarkets		____	____	____	____
10. Odor of dry goods stores and clothing departments		____	____	____	____
11. Odor of formalin or formaldehyde		____	____	____	____
12. Odor of chlorinated water		____	____	____	____
13. Drinking of chlorinated water		____	____	____	____
14. Fumes of chlorine gas		____	____	____	____
15. Odor of Clorox and other hypochlorite bleaches		____	____	____	____
16. Fumes from sulfur processing plants		____	____	____	____
17. Fumes of sulfur dioxide		____	____	____	____

These miscellaneous questions may yield some important clues. For example, pesticides constitute one of the most serious threats to the population, and especially to the chemically susceptible portion of the population.

Some people do not know whether they react to common pesticides but do know that they react to the fruit and vegetable sections of supermarkets, which are often sprayed with insecticides. Or they may find that they shun these sections, without being able to give a definite reason for their behavior. Often this can be traced to the adverse health effects of the fumes there.

A positive answer to any of questions 3 through 11, indicating either a strong like or dislike, is among the most significant facts which can be elicited by the questionnaire. For many years, pesticides have constituted the crux of the chemical susceptibility problem. I testified to this effect in the Senate Pesticide Hearings, chaired by Senator Abraham Ribicoff (D–Conn.) in 1963. Since that time the problem has only grown worse.

What Is Your Reaction to the Following?

	Check One:		Neu-	Dis-	Made sick
		Like	tral	like	from
Pine					
1. Odor of Christmas trees & other indoor evergreen decorations		____	____	____	____
2. Odor of knotty pine interiors		____	____	____	____

	Check One:	Like	Neu-tral	Dis-like	Made sick from
3. Odor from sanding or working with pine or cedar woods		___	___	___	___
4. Odor of cedar-scented furniture polish		___	___	___	___
5. Odor of pine-scented household deodorants		___	___	___	___
6. Odor of pine-scented bath oils, shampoos, or soaps		___	___	___	___
7. Odor of turpentine or turpentine-containing paints		___	___	___	___
8. Fumes from burning pine cones or wood		___	___	___	___

Many chemically susceptible persons react to pine and pine products. This may seem strange, since pine is a natural substance, whereas the chemicals we have focused on are mainly synthetic laboratory products. As was previously indicated, the reason for this may be that hydrocarbon fuels are ultimately derived from great pine forests which were buried aeons ago and compressed into the liquid form we know today.

Classes of Drugs, or Drugs—Circle if Suspected   Name Others Not Listed

Analgesics	Adrenalin (epinephrine)	_____
Androgens	Aminophyllin	_____
Anesthetics, local	Aspirin (Bufferin, Empirin)	_____
Anesthetics, general	Barbiturates	_____
Antibiotics	Codeine	_____
Anticoagulants	Demerol	_____
Anticonvulsants	Ephedrine	_____
Antihistaminics	Ether	_____
Antispasmodics	Iodides	_____
Asthma remedies	Mineral Oil	_____
Diuretics	Morphine	_____
Estrogens	Novocaine	_____
Headache remedies	Penicillin	_____
Laxatives	Phenobarbital	_____
Opiates	Phenolphthalein	_____
Sedatives	Saccharine	_____
Steroids	Stilbestrol	_____
Tranquilizers	Sucaryl	_____
Vaccines	Sulfonamides	_____
Vitamins	Vaseline	_____

Many of these drugs contain cornstarch, corn sugar, flavorings, colorings, fillers (excipients), and other substances added to improve the texture, flavor, or shelf life of the product. The drugs themselves, or any one of these other ingredients, can be the source of allergic-type reactions.

Drugs Currently Being Used—Circle If Suspected

_____	_____	_____
_____	_____	_____
_____	_____	_____
Currently used Dentifrice	Currently used Mouthwash	Others
		_____
Currently used Cosmetics	(name brands, if possible)	
Deodorant _____	*For Women*	*For Men*
Toilet soap _____	Face Powder _____	Electric preshave
Shampoo _____	Dusting Powder _____	_____
Hand Lotion _____	Lipstick _____	After shaving lotion
Cold cream _____	Foundation cream _____	_____
Contraceptive _____	Nail polish _____	Hair Oil _____
_____	Perfume _____	_____
_____	Cologne _____	Others _____
_____	Mascara _____	_____
_____	Eyebrow pencil _____	_____
_____	Cold Wave _____	_____
	Permanent _____	
	Hair tint _____	
	Douche _____	

As we have explained, drugs constitute an important part of the overall chemical susceptibility problem, and many patients' problems can be traced to these items. Many other individuals have developed long-term reactions to cosmetics and scents, which may be used in an addictive manner. Such scents are not only potentially dangerous for the wearer, but can be a source of irritation and reactions in others.

Do you smoke . . . cigarettes _____	pipe _____	cigars_____
Age you started to smoke _____	Age you last quit smoking _____	
Was it difficult to stop? _____	Number of smokes per day _____	
What is your maximum weight? _____	Your present weight? _____	

Finally, patients are asked about their smoking habits. Smoking is a significant factor, not only because of its proven relationship to cancer, heart disease, and other ailments, but because of the equally demonstrable relationship between tobacco smoke and common allergic-type reactions.

It should be emphasized that in interpreting this questionnaire, either a positive or a negative reaction can be significant. In other words, if a person reports that he *likes* the odor of insecticide spray, this is as significant as a dislike or intense hatred of the same odor. (Often, as has been said, the same person will have both of these reactions at different stages of his illness.)

It would be convenient to be able to give a numerical score to these questions. This cannot easily be done, however, since a reaction to *any* of these substances can indicate a chemical-susceptibility problem, and a person can have reactions to a small number of items on the list (or even to one of them) and still be affected. Most commonly, however, a person exhibits a broader pattern of reactions, and this is often revealed by reviewing the list. Multiple reactions are the rule, especially in advanced cases.

Although all questions are significant, a few are more significant than others. For reasons which have been explained, the ability to detect natural gas is among the most important indicators of the chemical-susceptibility syndrome. So, too, are the reactions to pesticide sprays (including either insecticides or herbicides), gasoline fumes, plastics, foam rubber, and the various synthetic drugs.

A broad pattern of likes and dislikes for any of the above substances should be taken as a sign that further medical help is needed and that preventive measures should be instituted.

One further point needs to be made: many people discover that they have the chemical-susceptibility problem, but do not think that they have a food allergy problem. Others know they have a food problem but ignore the chemical problem. Almost always, however, they have *both*, with one being predominant.

As knowledge of this field of environmental health has increased over the last thirty years, it has become apparent that the chemical problem is the dominant aspect. If the chemical problem is uncontrolled, the food allergy problem may be made worse. Such patients tend to lose their tolerance for foods which they previously tolerated, or fail to gain tolerance after avoiding previously troublesome foods.

The Chemical Questionnaire is therefore of great importance to all allergic patients and to all people who wish to avoid either aspect of environmental disease.

20
Coping with Chemical Exposure

It is possible for the average person to take steps to protect himself from the chemical environment. Although the cases of chemical susceptibility described in this book are, naturally, the most extreme examples, it should be emphasized that this problem can eventually affect a great many people who are presently without any strong or obvious symptoms. It is therefore wise for everyone to take steps to avoid developing chemical susceptibility before it reaches the clinical stage.

Eliminating all potentially troublesome chemicals, plastics, and synthetic materials from one's life may seem like a hopeless task. Some people who seem to agree with the point of view expressed in this book still argue that controlling these chemicals is impossible, since one must "live in the twentieth century."

There are several fallacies in this fatalistic argument.

First of all, the unbridled use of petrochemicals is part of a particular historical phase and has not been a constant in human history, by any means. In fact, with the much publicized energy shortage, it seems likely that the throwaway use of petrochemical products will have to be curtailed for economic reasons. The need to find more efficient, and also more healthy, forms of energy and basic materials has become a matter of survival in many countries. Thus the trend is with, not against, environmentalism in the long run.

Second, the degree to which harmful products are allowed into the environment is subject, to some extent, to political pressure and control. Countries, states, and even cities vary greatly in their regulations on health and pollution. In the 1920s, for instance, New York and other cities banned the use of leaded gasoline within their borders. Later, leaded gasoline was deregulated, largely because of pressure from the automobile and gasoline interests. But it was phased out once more in the 1960s and 1970s, largely as the result of political pressure. Toxic and cancer-causing substances have been somewhat restricted by federal law through the 1958 Delaney Amendment, banning carcinogens from food, and the 1976 Toxic Substances Control Act. These measures would never have been enacted without a groundswell of public opinion in their favor.

As public awareness of the danger of the unbridled use of petrochemicals grows and as more and more chronically ill people trace their problems to the "safe" chemical environment, we can expect to see increasing political action to control this danger as well. Thus, on a national and international level, there is no reason for pessimism, provided that people become aware of the danger and take effective action.

On a more personal level, it is advisable for each individual to restrict and eliminate harmful chemical exposures in the home, the workplace, and the general environment. If a person has cause to suspect chemical susceptibility, or only wishes to prevent it from occurring, there are a number of effective changes which can be made.

The following ten suggestions are not all-inclusive. As one learns more about ecologic illness and individual responses to chemicals, it will be possible to augment or modify this list. The basic idea behind these ten proposals, however, is to cut down on exposure to unsuspected causes of chronic illness.

Natural Gas

First on the list is natural gas. The case of Ellen Sanders (Chap. 3) is an extreme example of what natural gas can do to susceptible people. Many more people are less dramatically, but just as insidiously, affected by this product.

The use of the word "natural" in this context is misleading. Natural gas comes from the earth, but by and large it has lain there, trapped, for millennia. It is only in the past century that man has tapped this resource and brought himself into physical contact with it. Thus, natural gas is highly *unnatural* as far as the human body is concerned—a substance with which the body has no physiological method of coping. Synthetic chemicals are also added to this "natural" product, such as the one used to give it its characteristic "skunky" odor.

A leaking gas line is, of course, a life-threatening hazard: each year over a thousand people die of gas poisoning in the home.[1] An equally serious threat, in my opinion, is posed by the day-in and day-out inhalation of minute quantities of this same poisonous substance by the chemically susceptible.

We have been convinced by skillful advertising and public relations that natural gas is not only natural, but "safe" and "clean." Yet studies at the University of California and elsewhere have shown that the carbon monoxide and nitrogen dioxide levels in a vented kitchen become as high as in Los Angeles during a smog attack, when an oven has been heated to 350°F. for one hour. If the kitchen does *not* have an exhaust fan, these levels climb to *three times* the Los Angeles smog level in the same period.[2] Few people would not be susceptible to such high levels of indoor air pollution.

There are individuals, however, who are kept in a perpetual state of illness by far lower levels of the same poisonous substances. The gas which emanates from normal pilot lights or escapes from a well-saturated stove is often the main source of a patient's illness.

Given a choice, then, everyone should choose an electric range over a gas range. The first rule of prevention in this field is to minimize one's exposure to utility gas.

Since changing the stove might very well entail some expense, it is advisable to test oneself for reactions to the gas range first. This can be done by temporarily removing the range from the house, if at all possible. (A shut-off stove is better than a connected one but still disseminates gas into the environment.) Electric appliances such as a hot plate can be substituted for the range while the test is under way.

After the gas stove has been removed for a week or so, it can then be returned. The reader should keep a symptom diary, in which changes (positive or negative) in his condition can be noted. Both the removal of the gas stove and its reintroduction may be accompanied by changes in health. In cases in which the stove is definitely incriminated as a cause of symptoms, it should be permanently removed.

Although there may be some expense involved in making this change, it is a worthwhile investment in health. Several thousand patients have been guided in removing their gas ranges on the basis of such positive tests and not one has complained about the cost or reported being dissatisfied with the change.

No Smoking, Please!

If you smoke, it is necessary to quit in order to control environment chemical pollution. Making extensive changes in the home environment makes little sense if the individual insists on polluting himself and his living space with tobacco fumes. Nonsmokers and ex-smokers must get used to demanding breathing space in their own houses and in public places.

In uncooperative environments, the chemically susceptible person must stake a claim to part of the house as an off-limit, no-smoking oasis. The reason for this is that smoking is not only a major source of cancer, heart disease, and lung disease, but also an ecological disaster for the susceptible person.

Cigarette smoke is no simple thing: it contains hundreds of different chemicals, not all of which have been thoroughly analyzed. For example, tobacco, like other crops, is intensively sprayed with pesticides, and these are incompletely removed from the leaf before curing and packaging. When you breathe in someone else's tobacco smoke, you have the privilege of breathing in stale pesticide residues as well. Tobacco is frequently kept warm, while being cured in large barns, by kerosene-fueled heaters.[3] This kerosene, in trace amounts, then gets into the leaf and cannot be removed: it is present in the smoke as well. Each manufacturer adds flavor and taste additives which are composed of synthetic chemicals. These too are breathed in by the susceptible person, often perpetuating reactions to other common pollutants. The exact nature of these additives is guarded as a trade secret.

The cigarette smoker thus contaminates his own body and that of everyone around him.

There is still much to be learned about the hazards of cigarette consumption, hazards the $18 billion tobacco industry is not about to reveal. For example, in certain cases, cigarette smoke alone has been sufficient to cause schizophrenic-type reactions. One schizophrenic patient was able to control her symptoms with comprehensive food and chemical control. She then suddenly, and unexpectedly, suffered a relapse. Her bewildered parents finally discovered that when their daughter suffered such an attack, their son was in the room across the hall smoking a forbidden cigarette. In a comprehensive study conducted at the Fuller Memorial Sanitarium, South Attleboro, Massachusetts, Dr. William H. Philpott, director of research, and Dr. Marshall Mandell, showed that 75 percent of the patients who were classified as schizophrenics suffered mental symptoms from cigarette smoke. In fact, says Mandell, "tobacco smoke caused psychotic behavior in one out of ten."[4]

Since one food or chemical addiction feeds and supports another, bringing the total environment under control is the best way to beat the smoking habit.

Look Under the Sink!

Synthetic chemicals are found throughout the environment, but especially in home janitorial supplies. To rid the house of unnecessary air pollutants, start by looking under the sink. One can usually find there an accumulation of chemical products of all kinds: paints, solvents, laundry and dishwashing detergents, waxes and polishes, insect sprays, turpentine, shoe polish, and so forth. Whatever is not absolutely necessary should be dispensed with. Essential items, such as detergents, should be transferred to glass bottles with tight-fitting caps. One should save bottles for such a purpose. All questionable items should be stored outside, in places such as a garage or storeroom.

The same rule applies, naturally, to any other area in which toxic products accumulate. Conduct a careful house search, cleaning out drawers, broom closets, hobby areas, and medicine chests. It is amazing how much dangerous junk piles up in a house over the years, silently polluting the environment. One should be careful, however, not to allow any of these items to spill as they are being disposed of, or this may precipitate an acute attack of symptoms in susceptible people.

The human nose is an extraordinary instrument. Ecology patients tend to be either acutely sensitive to smells, or, conversely, lacking in the sense of smell altogether (in advanced cases). If you have a good-to-excellent sense of smell, you can identify noxious smells in the house by going out for a brisk walk in an area with fairly clean air and then returning to your house to perform a quick "sniff" test. If something has an offensive odor, *get rid of it*. Do not wait a day, or even a minute, since the nose will quickly adapt to the ill-smelling item. After being exposed for a short while, one can no longer fully smell the offending odor. Many patients report a cleaner feeling in the air after they have rid their homes of these hidden pollutants.

Several engineers and otherwise qualified experts now make "house calls" to inspect the homes of patients for chemical contaminants. They bring not only their expertise, but exceptional ability in "sniffing out" danger spots for patients, based on their own chemical-susceptibility problems. (The organizations listed in Appendix C can provide names of such experts.)

Reexamine Your Heating System

How to heat a home according to sound, ecologic principles is a topic beyond the scope of this book (see "Suggested Reading"). However, certain basic guidelines can be given to those responsible for this area of domestic life. First, it is a good idea to have a heating engineer recheck the efficiency and safety of the heating system periodically. This will minimize undetected leaks or breaks in the system and save money, as well as trips to the doctor.

If a chemically susceptible person has a gas-fired heating system, he has to consider changing it, or changing houses, regardless of the immediate cost. The reason is that it is difficult for a susceptible person to remain in anything resembling good health if he is subjected to the fumes of such a system.

An oil-fired heating system may also present a danger, since the fumes of the oil and its combustion products can often make their way into the living quarters of the house. If the oil is accidentally spilled, it is almost impossible ever to remove it, and fumes and odors will continue to contaminate the vicinity of the burner and beyond.

The ideal solution is to remove the heating unit from the house and locate it in a separate area or building of its own, so that only the hot water pipes enter the house. Installing electric heat, with or without solar heat, is another alternative.

For those in apartment houses who have a choice, it is best to live as far from the boiler room as possible. Steam or hot water radiators, on floors other than the ground level, are fairly good ecologically. It is a good idea to clean the radiators periodically and to give them an especially thorough cleaning in the fall before the heat is turned on.

Avoid Plastics

Plastic has become increasingly common, one might say all-pervasive, since the end of World War Two. The chemically susceptible person, however, should try to avoid unnecessary exposure to plastics wherever possible. The sources of plastics are explored in Chapter 6. As a simple preventive measure, one should go through one's house and make all obvious and necessary changes.

For example, many lamps now have plastic shades. As the light bulb heats up, the plastic begins to give off odors and fumes which can have a marked effect on mental and physical well-being. It is necessary, in such cases, to replace the plastic shades with shades made from glass, metal, or natural fabric. In the kitchen, plastic bowls and dishes should be replaced by ceramic, glass, or wooden ones. Wrap foods in aluminum foil instead of plastic wrap and use glass or metal containers instead of plastic refrigerator ware.

The degree to which one must make such changes obviously depends on the severity of the problem. Some people are able to tolerate the harder plastics, while others find they must make a clean sweep through the house in order to feel reasonably well. It is beyond the scope of this book to discuss every aspect of this large problem, although books listed in the "Suggested Reading" should be of help with the practical details.

Be Careful About Cars

Automobiles represent an important source of environmental problems. It has been pointed out in the case of Nora Barnes and other patients that some individuals react to even supposedly "harmless" amounts of automotive exhaust fumes (Chaps. 3 and 7). For this reason, the consumer should think ecologically when buying an automobile. There are five basic rules to follow when purchasing a car:

1. The car should have a valve which turns off the air intake. This is important, since one may run into unexpected sources of fumes on the road: a garbage dump, freshly tarred road, airport, driving through tunnels or unusually heavy traffic.
2. Choose the car upholstery with forethought. The best kind of upholstery

is leather, although this has become very difficult to find in American cars. The next best choice is rayon, a fabric made from cellulose, itself a wood by-product. Nylon is less objectionable than the newer synthetic fabrics such as vinyl.

3. The car should have push-button windows, to allow the driver to simultaneously raise all the windows when approaching a major source of pollution.

4. All rubber mats should be removed from the floor of the car and the trunk and should be replaced with carpeting, preferably made from natural fibers.

5. The car should be equipped with an activated carbon filter to clean up fumes which have accumulated on the inside. This is particularly important for those who are known to have a moderate-to-severe form of chemical susceptibility. Sources for such filters are given in the Golos book.

In general, one should be most careful when purchasing a car. It should be driven on the highway first, to see if unpleasant health symptoms develop when riding in it. There may be an undetected leak in the exhaust system, and any prepurchase inspection should pay careful attention to this part of the automobile. The car should preferably be tried out on a sunny, warm day, for plastic car upholstery can cause problems when heated. One should never buy a car which is a source of environmental problems or which causes or perpetuates symptoms.

Once a car is purchased, it is necessary and important to keep car fumes out of the living quarters. If there is a choice, avoid a house whose garage is located under or adjacent to the living area. The case of Sister Francesca, who fell asleep after being exposed to fumes from a still-hot car engine, illustrates the potential for reactions.

Detached garages are best. If the car must be stored in an adjacent garage, it should be allowed to cool completely, away from the house, before it is put away.

In choosing a house site, one should make sure that it is not located too close to any major road or highway, especially one on which busses travel. The direction of the prevailing winds should be taken into account as well. Check to find out if a new highway is planned for the neighborhood. Patients sometimes choose an ideal country spot for building an ecologically sound house, only to wake one morning to the sound of highway-building equipment.

Prepare a Bedroom Oasis

Everyone who is at all susceptible to chemicals needs at least one place to retreat to when he is at home. This is a place in which even the sickest chemical victim can feel relatively well and a base from which to plan future environmental changes. Dr. Guy O. Pfeiffer has called such a place an "oasis" within the polluted world.

The best place to construct such an oasis is a bedroom, preferably a small one. This can be converted into an ecologically sound haven. It must be thoroughly stripped and redecorated in order to prevent or minimize chemical problems.

First, all unnecessary items should be removed. The fewer things in the room the better. If there is a desk in the room, it should be placed somewhere else in the house. All books and magazines except those currently in use should be removed. (Some patients cannot even tolerate fresh reading material, because of the solvent-saturated ink used in printing.) All perfumes, scented powders, cosmetics, and lotions should be put elsewhere.

If there is carpeting in the room, it should also be removed or stored. The same holds for carpet pads, especially if they are made of foam rubber. The floors should either be bare wood or else should be covered by scatter rugs made from natural materials, such as wool or untreated cotton.

Cast a suspicious eye on all remaining furniture in the oasis. Has the dresser ever been put into storage? If it has, there is a good chance it was sprayed with pesticides. Does any of the furniture have a plastic coating? Has it recently been varnished, painted, or waxed? Use your senses, especially your nose, which is nature's built-in chemical detector, and ask others to do the same. Anything that smells unpleasant, offensive, or—literally—sickening may be the cause of chronic symptoms and should be removed from the oasis. Get rid of plastic venetian blinds as well, and synthetic curtain materials. Oil paintings should be moved, and plastic-framed pictures should be replaced with metal- and glass-framed pictures.

The closet in this bedroom oasis should be thoroughly cleaned out. All household chemicals, tools, hobby materials, shoe polishes, and other such items that may have accumulated on shelves or on the floor should be removed. Shelf paper, which may be impregnated with insect spray, should be thoroughly removed. Clothing in the closet, as well as that actually worn, should be restricted to garments made from natural materials. The closet door should close firmly, and some aluminum-foil barriers can be placed on the bottom of the door if there is a gap between the door itself and the floorboards. (There often is, since doors are now usually cut to anticipate plush carpeting.) Suitcases, camping gear, and the like should be stored elsewhere in the house.

The air conditioner can be an unexpected source of fumes. If the filter has been saturated with motor oil, it should be discarded and replaced with an unoiled filter which can then be treated with a vegetable oil to which you are not allergic.

Make sure no natural gas-heated air, or forced air, enters the room. The best solution is to shut off all outside sources of nonelectric heat and use a portable electric heater. This can be left at a low, nonfan setting, and it will generally produce enough heat to keep a small room at comfortable temperatures.

Since the average person spends eight hours a day in bed, it is obvious that this essential piece of furniture should be ecologically sound. First, get rid of any form of rubber pillows and substitute either a down pillow, if it is tolerated, or a cotton bedspread, which can be rolled up and placed in a cotton pillowcase to make an ecologically acceptable pillow.

The mattress should also have cotton stuffing. This is difficult to find, but one can cover a conventional mattress and bedsprings with zippered cotton covers. (Cotton/polyester covers are usually tolerated but pure cotton is superior.) These covers serve as barriers against synthetic fumes from foam rubber or fibers of petroleum origin. On top of the mattress, with its cover, one can put two cotton pads, and then cover them with cotton sheets. Blankets, likewise, should be made of natural fibers. Wool is best, if it is tolerated. If not, thermal cotton blankets are also available. Covering mattress with aluminum foil may help.

In the oasis, one will probably want a radio, television, and telephone. It is sometimes possible to get the telephone company to install an old-fashioned, hard-plastic Bakelite phone of the type that was common in the 1930s and 1940s. Bakelite radios can sometimes be found in used-furniture or antique stores. They are potentially less troublesome that those made of the softer modern plastics. Televisions often give off odors when hot, especially from the plastic-coated wires. There is no easy way around this difficulty. Try applying the "sniff test" to any television (after it has been playing for an hour or so) to see if it creates problems. Or try eliminating television entirely from this special room, if you wish.

You may hesitate to make such a radical change in lifestyle or be afraid that the oasis will be an eyesore. It need not be, for with its natural-fiber rugs on bare wooden floors, cheerful furniture and lamps, attractive curtains, and spare modern look, it may be aesthetically more pleasing than the room in its original state.

The most important question, of course, is the effect such an environment has on one's health. If you find, after spending a minimum of eight hours a day in this room for a week or two, that there is an improvement in chronic health symptoms, you may want to extend this style of living to other rooms in the house. When others see how well you feel, they will most probably cooperate in this project. Eventually, it is possible for the whole house to become an oasis for the entire family, which is what it was intended to be from the beginning—a place of true shelter. The unconscious introduction of various questionable substances into this household environment changed a shelter into a source of problems and danger. It is never too late to change it back again.

Working on the Workplace

Once the home oasis is established, it is possible to attempt to make changes in the workplace as well. If the patient is self-employed, this is usually fairly easy to arrange. If he or she works for someone else, it may require some argument to convince an employer to make changes for the patient's benefit. Sometimes it is easier to seek a transfer within a company or even another job which is less harmful to one's health.

In some cases, however, employers have been impressed enough with the change in an employee's health, including increased productivity, to voluntarily make ecologic changes in the workplace. After all, it is in their long-range interests, too, to have more productive employees. In some cases, employers have eventually come in as patients after seeing this method bring about improvements in the life of an employee.

Naturally, some polluted workshops are almost beyond repair for the ecology patient. In such cases, patients can take their health grievances to their unions or to the appropriate government agencies for adjustment.

Organic Diet

If all of the above changes have been made, and the chronic illness still has not been sufficiently improved, the patient should try eating a diet composed entirely of organic foods for two weeks. Preferably this should be the Rotary Diversified Diet described in Chapter 18.

It would be ideal if every person could eat organic food all the time. This is impossible to advocate today, since the supply of truly organic food of high quality is severely limited. Unsprayed, uncontaminated food should be made available first of all to those people who simply *cannot function without it*—the patients in advanced stages of chemical susceptibility.

An increasing demand for organic, uncontaminated food, however, should eventually lead to an increased supply of products. Consumers should be aware, however, that what passes for "organic" and "natural" nowadays is often not very pure, and susceptible patients often have reactions to what are at best semi-organic products.

A Constructive Point of View

It is important for anyone undertaking this program of prevention to maintain a constructive point of view. These problems are predominantly physical and external in origin, yet to the extent that psychological factors come into play, it is important to maintain a positive attitude. The necessary changes in lifestyle should be made of one's own free will, since no one such as a parent, spouse, or business associate can really make such important decisions for another person. At some point they must be self-motivated. Second, the patient should not be excessively sorry for himself. Anyone can learn to live a relatively healthy life in a less polluted environment. Despite the temporary difficulties, life can be made simpler and more enjoyable for the susceptible person. The aid and comfort of patients who have brought their own problems under control can be of great assistance.

These suggestions are offered as proposals for improving your health by changing the physical environment. They are not a panacea. Some people may need intensive care by a clinical ecologist or even temporary hospitalization before any real improvement is seen. For the most part, however, following these ten suggestions can make a big dent in a longstanding health problem, ward off any future cumulative chemical exposures, and help one to have a happier, safer, and more carefree existence.

IV
CONCLUSIONS

21
Clinical Ecology Versus Conventional Medicine

If money could buy health, America would be the healthiest country on earth. Per-capita spending on health care was $550 per person in 1976 and has been increasing rapidly since then. People over sixty-five spent three times that amount. Over $70 billion was disbursed at seven thousand hospitals in 1978. The cost of maintaining a mental patient rose to well over $13,000 per year.[1] Yet health—real health—continues to elude us. We spend more and more, and seem to get sicker and sicker.

We are all familiar with the frightening and well-publicized diseases, such as cancer, heart and circulatory ailments, and schizophrenia. Yet millions of people are sick in less visible, less obvious ways. Vast numbers of people are presently having their lives ruined by ill health but never make it into the health statistics. These are the chronically ill who suffer from combinations of perplexing symptoms. Some of these people either make the rounds from doctor to doctor, from old therapy to new, looking for an answer to their ill-defined medical problems, or become dropouts from a medical system which has done nothing but malign them; they have abandoned the orthodox approach but have found no viable alternative.

Often such patients are thrown into that convenient medical wastebasket, the psychiatric category. According to one government official, ten percent of the American public is in urgent need of psychiatric or psychological care. Ten percent—22 million people! In 1975, there were over 6.4 million "patient care episodes" in America's mental health facilities, with over 400,000 admissions to mental hospitals.[2] Most of us have the impression that such hospitals have diminished in importance over the years. Actually, although the *length of stay* has certainly decreased, the *number of admissions* has not: it is double what it was in 1960.

Between ten and thirty percent of all schoolchildren (depending on the study) are characterized as hyperactive.[3] This problem has been called the "single most common disorder seen by child psychiatrists." Often, such children are given drugs such as methylphenidate hydrochloride (Ritalin) to calm them down. Other studies claim that millions of children in the United States are mentally ill.[4]

Depression is now so widespread that it has been called "the common cold of mental disturbances." Suicide is a major source of death. Perhaps as many as two million persons attempt to kill themselves each year. At least 27,500 succeed—and statistics in this area notoriously understate the case.[5] Twenty million people suffer from manic-depressive disease.[6] Two million are victims of schizophrenia.[7] Six million are classified as retarded.[8] These are some of the "serious" mental health problems.

Countless other people, though, suffer in silence from what could be called cerebral symptoms. In one year—in 1964—a survey was conducted of people who suffered from headache, and it was found that about 24 million people consulted their physicians for this problem—about an eighth of the total population at that time. About half of these patients had migraines, the worst form of headache. The sales of aspirin and other pain relievers (about $600 million in 1977) testifies to the scope of this problem.[10]

Fatigue is so common that it is impossible to quantify. One doctor has estimated that 50 percent of all patients admitted to general hospitals in the United States list fatigue as one of their major complaints.[11] Addiction and drug abuse are so widespread that *Consumer Reports* states: ". . . the *nonuse* of mind-affecting drugs can be described as aberrant behavior, deviating from the norms of American society."[12]

So far, we have been looking mainly at cerebral problems. But in almost any area, the health statistics are alarming. A conventional allergist, for example, tried to tally the number of allergy patients in the country. (By "allergy" he meant only those diseases, such as hay fever and hives, which clinical ecologists would call minus-one or possibly minus-two withdrawal reactions.) He found that *half of the entire population* suffered from some form of allergy. Between eleven and twenty-two percent had "a really major allergy of serious, crippling proportions and consequences."[13]

Asthma and hay fever, both allergic in origin, rank third in prevalence among all chronic diseases. Asthma handicaps almost a million-and-a-half Americans and kills almost 2,000 people every year.[14]

Other conditions which have been linked to environmental problems are equally crippling. Thirty million people in the United States, or almost one in seven, are officially listed as handicapped. Arthritis and rheumatism top the list of causes, but heart conditions, hypertension, diabetes, and muscle problems all contributed.[15]

It should be clear, then, that the conventional approach to this mass of health problems is not working well. The growing health-consumer rebellion is largely a result of the inability of orthodox medicine to treat conditions which, frequently, are more easily and properly prevented through environmental controls. In almost any area of chronic illness, the failure of conventional medicine is conspicuous, and nowhere more so than in so-called psychiatric disorders.

Psychiatry has a special relationship to clinical ecology, since usually allergy patients have been misdiagnosed as neurotics and psychotics by well-meaning but misinformed physicians. Yet few of the treatment strategies of psychiatry have lived up to their promise. Since I began practicing medicine over forty years ago, I have seen, one after another, psychoanalysis, lobotomy, electroshock therapy, and drug therapy each overestimated by enthusiastic proponents. Each one raised the hopes of so-called mental patients and their families, each had well-publicized successes but many unpublicized failures as well. Drugs which affect the central nervous system are now a $2.2 billion business (not counting illicit drugs).[16] These may tranquilize, stimulate, or ease the mind into oblivion, but in general they do not get at the root cause of a person's problem. And they themselves may cause illness, not the least of which is the chemical-susceptibility problem.

It would be an easy task to emphasize the failings of psychiatry by pointing out the welter of faddish therapies which have succeeded the now widely questioned methods of strict Freudian psychoanalysis: transactional analysis, hypnotherapy, family therapy, primal screaming, EST, rebirthing, rolfing, and so on. It would be equally easy to point to the false hopes and promises of cures which marked the history of psychiatric treatment.

The same could be said about other medical fields, including the specialty of allergy. The critical point, however, is not simply to castigate the orthodox medical profession, but to understand how it has gotten itself so boxed in and how this situation can be changed. One thing is clear: the crisis of American medicine did not begin recently but has its roots in medical history and in the general history of Western science. It is a one-sided overgrowth of certain features of Western medicine which has resulted in both its most conspicuous successes and its worst limitations and failures.

In the seventeenth century, the French philosopher René Descartes suggested that scientists leave the mind out of their considerations of biology and focus instead on the workings of the body. Descartes compared the physical body to a machine and suggested that it could be analyzed section by section, in increasingly minute detail. In this way, he thought, scientists could reach ultimate truths about the nature of life.

This was the technique of analysis which always sought to reduce the complex to the simple in all of its deliberations. Analysis has remained the dominant approach to biological problems since then, to the virtual exclusion of more well-rounded, holistic approaches.

This overly analytical approach has had several unfortunate consequences. For one thing, it contributed to the dichotomy, or split, between mental and physical symptoms which continues to this day. The "scientific" physician dealt only with physical problems, and sent so-called mental problems to a special kind of healer called a psychiatrist. The organic link between mind and body was not grasped.

Second, the analytical scientist could not see man as part of nature and as a dynamic creature constantly acting upon—and being acted upon by—his physical and social environment. A cadaver could be dissected, but a living man or woman had to be considered in his real environment. This the analytical school could not do. Instead, undue emphasis was put on the anatomical features of a person's illness, which often revealed little or nothing about the environmental source of the problem. In fact, the word "cause," in conventional terminology, came to mean "physical mechanisms" within the body itself, rather than environmental causes.

Third, the analysts sought uniform laws to explain all bodily phenomena. But this textbook approach often failed to take into account the individual nature of a patient's illness, an individualism which results from the subtle differences that exist between people, as well as the different environmental factors which affect their health. Medicine became mass-produced and thereby missed the unique aspects of each person's illness.

Using analytical techniques, the conventional physician cannot find the environmental causes of a patient's chronic illness; he usually does not even get close. Yet since treatment is called for, he resorts to methods which attempt to alter or coverup *symptoms*. For headaches or for arthritis he prescribes pain-killers. For hyperactivity in children, Ritalin. For depression, the tricyclic drugs. For manic-depressive disease, lithium chloride.

Some of these techniques have undeniable relief value, but often they cause more problems than they help. In all cases, however, they are not based on a fundamental knowledge of individual environmental causes. Thus the failure of conventional medicine to successfully treat chronic illness is not a superficial problem caused by a mere lack of information. It is a failure fundamental to the analytical bias of most Western science.

By contrast, psychiatrists often do attempt to understand the environmental origins of their patients' illnesses. The problem here is that they confine the meaning of "environment" largely to *interpersonal relations*. In my experience, interpersonal difficulties are rarely the cause of mental disturbances. Rather, the personal kind of problems are side effects of the same underlying problem which is causing depression, hyperactivity, alcoholism, or other signs of so-called mental disease: that is, in most cases, a maladaptation to the *nonpersonal*, or material, environment.

The psychiatric approach may cause unnecessary harm. Its methods are sometimes devastating to family and social ties, which are absolutely basic to the recovery of patients with mental disturbances. In a typical case, the patient blames some family member, friend, or associate for his problem. Actually, this person is only an innocent bystander drawn into the tumultuous aftertow of an environmental reaction. When the patient targets the friend or family member, however, this disturbed interpersonal realtionship may become an established part of his story. The patient, in other words, has found a scapegoat. These "insights" of the patient are then constantly repeated to the psychiatrist, psychologist, family physician, clergyman, or other willing listener. Sooner or later, some professionals may agree with the patient's "insights" or suggest a trial separation based on this erroneous idea.

Just at the time when the disturbed person needs his friends and family the most, he may be deprived of their support, sometimes with the connivance of members of the medical profession. The innocent bystander understandably blames the professionals for being homewreckers. The professional, however, is only accepting the patient's heartfelt (but erroneous) explanation of his problem, which fits the psychiatrist's own theory of chronic illness.

The pattern of incriminating some innocent bystander is then almost invariably repeated in the next social setting. A new "scapegoat" must and will be found, for the seriously ill patient, in the midst of an inexplicable reaction, lashes out at those around him as he desperately seeks to make sense out of his difficulties. This process of "scapegoating" is a downward spiral, by which many victims of environmentally induced illnesses lose their moral and material support just when they need it the most.

To summarize, then, for many people with chronic illnesses of all sorts, the medical system has become a frustrating rat race, an expensive, exhausting maze from which there appears to be no escape. Many doctors are equally frustrated, but see no viable alternative.

The net result has been a crisis of unprecedented proportions in American medicine, a loss of hope amidst once undreamed-of technology, and a growing sense of discontent and rebellion.

There is real tragedy here, for in fact many people with chronic illnesses *can* be helped. A vast, although still undetermined, number of them are suffering from nothing more than a maladaptation to their environment. This maladaptation to corn, wheat, coffee, and other common foods, or to natural gas, or to chemical pollutants, is ever-present, ongoing, and subtle, so that its nature is rarely even glimpsed by the victim. It is certainly a tragedy to see such a person shunted from specialist to specialist, none of whom knows any more about his problem than he does—operated upon, maligned, drugged, alienated from friends and family—when all the time his problem was no more mysterious than an intolerance to avoidable foods and pollutants.

Yet such patients can get better, feel well, and lead productive lives. The population as a whole could experience a tremendous increase in well-being and productivity if food and chemical susceptibility were routinely considered in each case of chronic disease, just as infection is today.

How has it happened, then, that this topic is so unknown?

First, there is the hidden nature of the disease. Microbial infections were only dimly suspected until the invention of the microscope. After that it became possible for scientists and even laymen to incriminate germs in the origin of diseases, mostly acute illnesses. Food and chemical susceptibility were likewise unsuspected until the discovery of new diagnostic techniques for unmasking them. The average person, and even the average physician, is still unaware of the prevalence of these allergies in causing chronic illness. Thus, innocently, the victim of this problem goes on perpetuating it for months and years.

Second, since the problem involves an addictive phase, there is an unconscious tendency to protect the source of the problem from exposure. Living and eating habits are routinely designed to feed addictions, not to break them. In the face of a barrage of advertising, food addicts and "junk-food junkies" shut their ears to the truth about their favorite foods. In addition, we have been conditioned to accept our new plastic environment as the hallmark of "progress," and each shiny new convenience as a big step forward. These conveniences are highly inconvenient, however, if they lead to increased illness and decreased health, energy, and happiness.

Third, we have had to contend with the disinterest, if not the ignorance, of much of the medical profession about this topic. The growth of medical specialization in this century has created a highly unnatural situation in which each physician is more or less concerned with one part of the body, with little attention paid to the whole person. The medical profession has been largely uncomfortable with synthetic (unifying) concepts. Specialization has turned out to be a convenient and, of course, lucrative way of dividing the labors of medicine. Most physicians have therefore neglected holistic approaches to medicine, such as clinical ecology, which do not seem to fit into neatly compartmentalized categories.

Allergists seemingly should be more receptive, since allergy too deals with many different anatomical sites: it is more holistic than, say, gastroenterology. There are special difficulties here, though. For one thing, allergists already feel overwhelmed by the task of treating conventional allergic reactions, such as hay fever and asthma. There are only about 1,300 allergists in the United

States to care for over 100 million people with such problems. They are kept busy, since allergy patients also require three times as many office visits as those with other types of illnesses. Conventional allergy treatments for inhalants (pollens, dust, molds, and so forth) work reasonably well, and most allergists are therefore content to spend their time treating an ample supply of such patients. There is little practical impetus for them to do otherwise.

It bears repeating that on a theoretical level American allergists were induced by their European counterparts, in 1925, to redefine the field in terms of antibodies and antigens. Since many inhalant allergies do create distinctive antibodies in the blood, this seemed like a reasonable thing to do. As time went on, however, new types of "allergies" were discovered, specifically those discussed in this book. These "allergies" apparently did not work by conventional means. Instead of changing the definition to include the new phenomena, the leaders of the field chose instead to stick with their outmoded definitions and to minimize the significance of the new scientific evidence.

A final factor is industry. Clinical ecology is conspicuously independent of industrial influence. Patients of conventional allergists and chest doctors spend over $100 million on injections, over $50 million on antihistamines, and contribute much of the $170 million spent on bronchial dilators.[17]

Clinical ecology patients spend almost nothing on such commodities. The reason is, of course, that clinical ecology urges patients to shun drugs, whenever possible, and rely instead on the avoidance of incriminated substances. Therefore clinical ecology has not been the beneficiary of any largesse from the drug industry, as many conventional fields have been, nor has it received any money from the government or large foundations. Those who believe in the drug approach have not taken kindly to this philosophy.

Our approach also stresses the avoidance of various commonly eaten foods or at least a decrease in their habitual consumption. Most of these foods, as we have mentioned, form the basis of huge industries. This fact is also unlikely to win us powerful allies in the consumer society. At many junctures we have faced active obstruction and opposition from industrial interests—such as, for instance, the corn products industry. It does not please this industry to hear that corn, one of the most prevalent foods in the American diet, is the leading cause of food addiction. People will inevitably use corn and its by-products more judiciously as this fact becomes better known.

There are obviously good reasons, then, why clinical ecology has faced an uphill battle. Through books such as this one, however, information about the new system is finally being put in the hands of those who need it. It is now up to the public, in concert with concerned physicians and professionals, to bring about the necessary changes. It may seem strange for a physician to call on laypeople to make medical changes. But fifty years of experience have demonstrated to me that the medical profession itself will not take the necessary steps. It remains for the public to act in its own interest and convince doctors of the need for a new and more fundamentally sound approach to chronic illness.

There is ample precedent for this. In the nineteenth century, public involvement in the Popular Health Movement and other such groups led to better sanitation, living standards, and health education.[18] At the beginning of this century, it was again the public which fought the uncontrolled spread of fraudulent patent medicines and the unhygienic practices of the food industries. This led to the passage, in 1906, of the epoch-making Food and Drug Act.[19] More recently, it has mainly been laypeople who have strugged for a cleaner environment and a healthier workplace. A decade of public education and agitation culminated in Earth Day, 1970, widely observed by practically everybody but the medical profession. These activities, in turn, prepared the way for the major environmental regulations of the 1970s, such as the Toxic Substances Control Act of 1976.

Clinical ecology has inherited and incorporated many of the features of these previous movements. It draws its inspiration from the fact that the public, once educated and aroused, can and will take the necessary steps to better health.

For millions of people, this alternative approach to healing cannot come too soon.

Appendix A
The Food Families

The following lists of food families can be used in constructing a Rotary Diversified Diet. In List 1, most commonly eaten foods are listed alphabetically. Each is preceded by the number of its food family. These same foods are then categorized by family in List 2. In this way, the reader can avoid eating foods from the same family group in a repetitive way. The lists are taken, with permission, from *Coping with Your Allergies* by Natalie Golos et al. (New York: Simon and Schuster, 1979). This was taken, in turn, largely from Alsoph H. Corwin: "The Rotary Diet and Taxonomy," Lawrence D. Dickey, ed., *Clinical Ecology* (Springfield, Illinois, Charles C Thomas, 1976), pp. 122–148.

LIST 1
FOOD FAMILIES (ALPHABETICAL)

A

81	abalone	54	althea root
80	absinthe	12	Amaryllis Family
41	acacia (gum)	94	amberjack
46	acerola	86	American eel
79	acorn squash	117	Amphibians
1	agar-agar	85	anchovy
12	agave	65	angelica
98	albacore	65	anise
41	alfalfa	38	annatto
1	Algae	136	antelope
63	allspice	40a	apple
40b	almond	73	apple mint
11	*Aloe vera*	40b	apricot
		47	arrowroot, Brazilian (tapioca)

223

111	carp	111	chub
29	Carpetweed Family	7	chufa
1	carrageen	40a	cider
65	carrot	34	cinnamon
65	Carrot Family	1	citric acid
79	casaba melon	45	citron
79	caserta squash	6	citronella
48	cashew	45	Citrus Family
48	Cashew Family	81	clam
47	cassava	73	clary
34	cassia bark	63	clove
47	castor bean	41	clover
47	castor oil	55	cocoa
88	catfish (ocean)	55	cocoa butter
112	catfish species	8	coconut
73	catnip	79	cocozelle
36	cauliflower	87	cod (scrod)
104	caviar	76	coffee
74	cayenne pepper	55	cola nut
65	celeriac	36	collards
65	celery	80	coltsfoot
80	celtuce	36	colza shoots
9	ceriman	71	comfrey
80	chamomile	80	Composite Family
52	champagne	5	Conifer Family
28	chard	65	coriander
79	chayote	6	corn
40b	cherry	78	corn-salad
65	chervil	80	costmary
24	chestnut	54	cottonseed oil
73	chia seed	41	coumarin
124	chicken	36	couve tronchuda
41	chickpea	41	cowpea
67	chicle	82	crab
80	chicory	40a	crabapple
74	chili pepper	66	cranberry
36	Chinese cabbage	114	crappie
56	Chinese gooseberry	82	crayfish
14	Chinese potato	52	cream of tartar
79	Chinese preserving melon	79	Crenshaw melon
7	Chinese water chestnut	96	croaker
24	chinquapin	79	crookneck squash
11	chives	79	cucumber
55	chocolate	65	cumin

6	grits
74	ground cherry
7	groundnut
91	grouper
123	grouse (ruffed)
63	guava
125	guinea fowl
41	gum acacia
41	gum tragacanth

H

87	haddock
87	hake
103	halibut
101	harvest fish
23	hazelnut
22	heartnut
66	Heath Family
54	hibiscus
22	hickory nut
134	hog
49	Holly Family
6	hominy
79	honeydew
77	Honeysuckle Family
25	hop
73	horehound
133	horse
36	horseradish
3	horsetail
3	Horsetail Family
79	Hubbard squash
66	huckleberry
73	hyssop

I

15	Iris Family
1	Irish moss

J

68	Japanese persimmon
80	Jerusalem artichoke
41	jicama
5	juniper

K

68	kaki
36	kale
1	kelp
41	kidney bean
56	kiwi berry
36	kohlrabi
45	kumquat

L

137	lamb
28	lamb's-quarters
34	Laurel Family
73	lavender
41	lecithin
11	leek
41	Legume Family
45	lemon
73	lemon balm
6	lemon grass
72	lemon verbena
41	lentil
80	lettuce
41	licorice
11	Lily Family
41	lima bean
45	lime
53	linden
53	Linden Family
51	litchi
82	lobster
40c	loganberry
40c	longberry
79	loofah
40a	loquat
65	lovage
79	*Luffa*
51	lychee

M

26	macadamia
33	mace
98	mackerel

124	peafowl
41	peanut
40a	pear
22	pecan
40a	pectin
75	Pedalium Family
73	pennyroyal
74	pepino
74	pepper, sweet
21	peppercorn
21	Pepper Family
73	peppermint
102	perch (ocean)
113	perch (white)
115	perch (yellow)
79	Persian melon
68	persimmon
124	pheasant
109	pickerel
122	pigeon (squab)
30	pigweed
109	pike
84	pilchard (sardine)
63	*Pimenta*
74	pimiento
10	pineapple
10	Pineapple Family
5	pine nut
21	*Piper*
48	pistachio
103	plaice
16	plantain
40b	plum
9	poi
48	poison ivy
87	pollack
61	pomegranate
61	Pomegranate Family
94	pompano
6	popcorn
35	Poppy Family
35	poppyseed
97	porgy
74	potato

74	Potato Family
82	prawn
79	preserving melon
60	prickly pear
26	Protea Family
40	prune
2	puffball
12	pulque
45	pummelo
79	pumpkin
114	pumpkinseed (sunfish)
30	purslane
30	Purslane Family
80	pyrethrum

Q

124	quail
18	Queensland arrowroot
26	Queensland nut
40	quince

R

129	rabbit
36	radish
52	raisin
11	ramp
36	rape
40	raspberry
119	rattlesnake
41	red clover
135	reindeer
118	Reptiles
27	rhubarb
6	rice
137	Rocky Mountain sheep
105	roe
80	romaine
40	Rose Family
102	rosefish
40	rosehips
54	roselle
73	rosemary
45	Rue Family
123	ruffed grouse

LIST 2
FOOD FAMILIES (NUMERICAL)

Plant

1 Algae
   agar-agar
   carrageen (Irish moss)
   *dulse
   kelp (seaweed)
2 Fungi
   baker's yeast ("Red Star")
   brewer's or nutritional yeast
   mold (in certain cheeses)
      citric acid *(Aspergillus)*
   morel
   mushroom
   puffball
   truffle
3 Horsetail Family, *Equisetaceae*
   *shavegrass (horsetail)
4 Cycad Family, *Cycadaceae*
   Florida arrowroot *(Zamia)*
5 Conifer Family, *Coniferae*
   *juniper (gin)
      pine nut (piñon, pinyon)
6 Grass Family, *Gramineae*
   barley
      malt
      maltose
   bamboo shoots
   corn (mature)
      corn meal
      corn oil
      cornstarch
      corn sugar
      corn syrup
      hominy grits
      popcorn
   lemon grass
      citronella
   millet
   oat
      oatmeal

rice
   rice flour
rye
sorghum grain
   syrup
sugarcane
   cane sugar
   molasses
   raw sugar
sweet corn
triticale
wheat
   bran
   bulgur
   flour
      gluten
      graham
      patent
      whole wheat
   wheat germ
wild rice
7 Sedge Family, *Cyperaceae*
   Chinese water chestnut
   chufa (groundnut)
8 Palm Family, *Palmaceae*
   coconut
      coconut meal
      coconut oil
   date
      date sugar
   palm cabbage
   sago starch *(Metroxylon)*
9 Arum Family, *Araceae*
   ceriman *(Monstera)*
   dasheen *(Colocasia)*
      arrowroot
   taro *(Colocasia)* arrowroot
      poi

* One or more plant parts (leaf, root, seed, etc.) used as a beverage.

malanga *(Xanthosoma)*
yautia *(Xanthosoma)*

10 Pineapple Family, *Bromeliaceae*
pineapple

11 Lily Family, *Liliaceae*
Aloe vera
asparagus
chives
garlic
leek
onion
ramp
*sarsaparilla
shallot
yucca (soap plant)

12 Amaryllis Family, *Amaryllidaceae*
agave
mescal, pulque, and tequila

13 Tacca Family, *Taccaceae*
Fiji arrowroot *(Tacca)*

14 Yam Family, *Dioscoreaceae*
Chinese potato (yam)
ñame (yampi)

15 Iris Family, *Iridaceae*
orris root (scent)
saffron *(Crocus)*

16 Banana Family, *Musaceae*
arrowroot *(Musa)*
banana
plantain

17 Ginger Family, *Zingiberaceae*
cardamon
East Indian arrowroot
(Curcuma)
ginger
turmeric

18 Canna Family, *Cannaceae*
Queensland arrowroot

19 Arrowroot Family, *Marantaceae*
arrowroot (*Maranta* starch)

20 Orchid Family, *Orchidaceae*
vanilla

21 Pepper Family, *Piperaceae*
peppercorn *(Piper)*
black pepper
white pepper

22 Walnut Family, *Juglandaceae*
black walnut
butternut
English walnut
heartnut
hickory nut
pecan

23 Birch Family, *Betulaceae*
filbert (hazelnut)
oil of birch (wintergreen)
(some wintergreen flavor is
methyl salicylate)

24 Beech Family, *Fagaceae*
chestnut
chinquapin

25 Mulberry Family, *Moraceae*
breadfruit
fig
*hop
mulberry

26 Protea Family, *Proteaceae*
macadamia (Queensland nut)

27 Buckwheat Family, *Polygonaceae*
buckwheat
garden sorrel
rhubarb
sea grape

28 Goosefoot Family, *Chenopodia-
ceae*
beet
chard
lamb's-quarters
spinach
sugar beet
tampala

29 Carpetweed Family, *Aizoaceae*
New Zealand spinach

30 Purslane Family, *Portulacaceae*
pigweed (purslane)

* One or more plant parts (leaf, root, seed, etc.) used as a beverage.

31 Buttercup Family, *Ranuncula-*
   ceae
   *golden seal
32 Custard-Apple Family
   Annona species
   custard-apple
   papaw (pawpaw)
33 Nutmeg Family, *Myristicaceae*
   nutmeg
   mace
34 Laurel Family, *Lauraceae*
   avocado
   bay leaf
   cassia bark
   cinnamon
   *sassafras
   filé (powdered leaves)
35 Poppy Family, *Papaveraceae*
   poppyseed
36 Mustard Family, *Cruciferae*
   broccoli
   Brussels sprouts
   cabbage
   cardoon
   cauliflower
   Chinese cabbage
   collards
   colza shoots
   couve tronchuda
   curly cress
   horseradish
   kale
   kohlrabi
   mustard greens
   mustard seed
   radish
   rape
   rutabaga (swede)
   turnip
   upland cress
   watercress
37 Caper Family, *Capparidaceae*
   caper

38 Bixa Family, *Bixaceae*
   annatto (natural yellow dye)
39 Saxifrage Family, *Saxifragaceae*
   currant
   gooseberry
40 Rose Family, *Rosaceae*
   a. *pomes*
      apple
         cider
            vinegar
            pectin
      crabapple
      loquat
      pear
      quince
      *rosehips
   b. *stone fruits*
      almond
      apricot
      cherry
      peach (nectarine)
      plum (prune)
      sloe
   c. *berries*
      blackberry
      boysenberry
      dewberry
      loganberry
      longberry
      youngberry
      *raspberry (leaf)
      black raspberry
      red raspberry
      purple raspberry
      *strawberry (leaf)
      wineberry
   d. *herb*
      burnet (cucumber flavor)
41 Legume Family, *Leguminoseae*
   *alfalfa (sprouts)
   beans
      fava
      lima
      mung (sprouts)
      navy
      string (kidney)

* One or more plant parts (leaf, root, seed, etc.) used as a beverage.

black-eyed pea (cowpea)
*carob
  carob syrup
chickpea (garbanzo)
*fenugreek
gum acacia
gum tragacanth
jicama
kudzu
lentil
*licorice
pea
peanut
  peanut oil
*red clover
*senna
soybean
  lecithin
  soy flour
  soy grits
  soy milk
  soy oil
tamarind
tonka bean
  coumarin

42 Oxalis Family, *Oxalidaceae*
carambola
oxalis

43 Nasturtium Family, *Tropaeolaceae*
nasturtium

44 Flax Family, *Linaceae*
*flaxseed

45 Rue (Citrus) Family, *Rutaceae*
citron
grapefruit
kumquat
lemon
lime
murcot
orange
pummelo
tangelo
tangerine

46 Malpighia Family, *Malpighiaceae*
acerola (Barbados cherry)

47 Spurge Family, *Euphorbiaceae*
cassava or yuca *(Manihot)*
  cassava meal
  tapioca (Brazilian
    arrowroot)
castor bean
  castor oil

48 Cashew Family, *Anacardiaceae*
cashew
mango
pistachio
poison ivy
poison oak
poison sumac

49 Holly Family, *Aquifoliaceae*
maté (yerba maté)

50 Maple Family
maple sugar
maple syrup

51 Soapberry Family, *Sapindaceae*
litchi (lychee)

52 Grape Family, *Vitaceae*
grape
  brandy
  champagne
  cream of tartar
  dried "currant"
  raisin
  wine
  wine vinegar
muscadine

53 Linden Family, *Tiliaceae*
*basswood (linden)

54 Mallow Family, *Malvaceae*
*althea root
cottonseed oil
*hibiscus (roselle)
okra

* One or more plant parts (leaf, root, seed, etc.) used as a beverage.

55 Sterculia Family, *Sterculiaceae*
    *chocolate (cacao)
    *cocoa
      cocoa butter
      cola nut
56 Dillenia Family, *Dilleniaceae*
    Chinese gooseberry (kiwi berry)
57 Tea Family, *Theaceae*
    *tea
58 Passion Flower Family, *Passiflora-ceae*
    granadilla (passion fruit)
59 Papaya Family, *Caricaceae*
    papaya
60 Cactus Family, *Cactaceae*
    prickly pear
61 Pomegranate Family, *Puniceae*
    pomegranate
      grenadine
62 Sapucaya Family, *Lecythidaceae*
    Brazil nut
    sapucaya nut (paradise nut)
63 Myrtle Family, *Myrtaceae*
    allspice *(Pimenta)*
    clove
    *eucalyptus
    guava
64 Ginseng Family, *Araliaceae*
    *American ginseng
    *Chinese ginseng
65 Carrot Family, *Umbelliferae*
    angelica
    anise
    caraway
    carrot
      carrot syrup
    celeriac (celery root)
    celery
    *seed & leaf
    chervil
    coriander
    cumin
    dill
      dill seed

    *fennel
      finocchio
        Florence fennel
    *gotu kola
    *lovage
    *parsley
    parsnip
    sweet cicely
66 Heath Family, *Ericaceae*
    *bearberry
    *blueberry
    cranberry
    *huckleberry
67 Sapodilla Family, *Sapotaceae*
    chicle (chewing gum)
68 Ebony Family, *Ebonaceae*
    American persimmon
    kaki (Japanese persimmon)
69 Olive Family, *Oleaceae*
    olive (green or ripe)
    olive oil
70 Morning-Glory Family, *Convol-vulaceae*
    sweet potato
71 Borage Family, *Boraginaceae* (Herbs)
    borage
    *comfrey (leaf & root)
72 Verbena Family, *Verbenaceae*
    *lemon verbena
73 Mint Family, *Labiatae* (Herbs)
    apple mint
    basil
    bergamot
    *catnip
    *chia seed
    clary
    *dittany
    *horehound
    *hyssop
    lavender
    *lemon balm
    marjoram

---

* One or more plant parts (leaf, root, seed, etc.) used as a beverage.

oregano
*pennyroyal
*peppermint
rosemary
sage
*spearmint
summer savory
thyme
winter savory
74 Potato Family, *Solanaceae*
  eggplant
  ground cherry
  pepino
    (melon pear)
  pepper (Capsicum)
    bell, sweet
    cayenne
    chili
    paprika
    pimiento
  potato
  tobacco
  tomatillo
  tomato
  tree tomato
75 Pedalium Family, *Pedaliaceae*
  sesame seed
    sesame oil
    tahini
76 Madder Family, *Rubiaceae*
  *
  woodruff
77 Honeysuckle Family, *Caprifoliaceae*
  elderberry
    elderberry flowers
78 Valerian Family, *Valerianaceae*
  corn salad (fetticus)
79 Gourd Family, *Cucurbitaceae*
  chayote
  Chinese preserving melon
  cucumber
  gherkin

loofah *(Luffa)* (vegetable
    sponge)
muskmelons
  cantaloupe
  casaba
  crenshaw
  honeydew
  Persian melon
pumpkin
  pumpkin seed & meal
squashes
  acorn
  buttercup
  butternut
  Boston marrow
  caserta
  cocozelle
  crookneck & straightneck
  cushaw
  golden nugget
  Hubbard varieties
  pattypan
  turban
  vegetable spaghetti
  zucchini
watermelon
80 Composite Family, *Compositae*
  *boneset
  *burdock root
  cardoon
  chamomile
  *chicory
  coltsfoot
  costmary
  dandelion
  endive
  escarole
  globe artichoke
  *goldenrod
  Jerusalem artichoke
    artichoke flour
  lettuce
    celtuce

* One or more plant parts (leaf, root, seed, etc.) used as a beverage.

pyrethrum
romaine
safflower oil
salsify (oyster plant)
santolina (herb)
scolymus (Spanish oyster plant)
scorzonera (black salsify)
southernwood

sunflower
   sunflower seed, meal, & oil
tansy (herb)
tarragon (herb)
witloof chicory (French endive)
wormwood (absinthe)
*yarrow

Animal

81 *Mollusks*
  Gastropods
    abalone
    snail
  Cephalopod
    squid
  Pelecypods
    clam
    cockle
    mussel
    oyster
    scallop

82 *Crustaceans*
  crab
  crayfish
  lobster
  prawn
  shrimp

83 *Fishes (saltwater)*

84 Herring Family
  menhaden
  pilchard (sardine)
  sea herring

85 Anchovy Family
  anchovy

86 Eel Family
  American eel

87 Codfish Family
  cod (scrod)
  cusk

  haddock
  hake
  pollack

88 Sea Catfish Family
  ocean catfish

89 Mullet Family
  mullet

90 Silverside Family
  silverside (whitebait)

91 Sea Bass Family
  grouper
  sea bass

92 Tilefish Family
  tilefish

93 Bluefish Family
  bluefish

94 Jack Family
  amberjack
  pompano
  yellow jack

95 Dolphin Family
  dolphin

96 Croaker Family
  croaker
  drum
  sea trout
  silver perch
  spot
  weakfish (spotted sea trout)

97 Porgy Family
  northern scup (porgy)

* One or more plant parts (leaf, root, seed, etc.) used as a beverage.

98 Mackerel Family
    albacore
    bonito
    mackerel
    skipjack
    tuna
99 Marlin Family
    marlin
    sailfish
100 Swordfish Family
    swordfish
101 Harvestfish Family
    butterfish
    harvestfish
102 Scorpionfish Family
    rosefish (ocean perch)
103 Flounder Family
    dab
    flounder
    halibut
    plaice
    sole
    turbot
104 *Fishes (freshwater)*
104 Sturgeon Family
    sturgeon (caviar)
105 Herring Family
    shad (roe)
106 Salmon Family
    salmon species
    trout species
107 Whitefish Family
    whitefish
108 Smelt Family
    smelt
109 Pike Family
    muskellunge
    pickerel
    pike
110 Sucker Family
    buffalofish

    sucker
111 Minnow Family
    carp
    chub
112 Catfish Family
    catfish species
113 Bass Family
    white perch
    yellow bass
114 Sunfish Family
    black bass species
    sunfish species
      pumpkinseed
    crappie
115 Perch Family
    sauger
    walleye
    yellow perch
116 Croaker Family
    freshwater drum
117 *Amphibians*
117 Frog Family
    frog (frogs legs)
118 Reptiles
119 Snake Family
    rattlesnake
120 Turtle Family
    terrapin
    turtle species
121 *Birds*
121 Duck Family
    duck
      eggs
    goose
      eggs
122 Dove Family
    dove
    pigeon (squab)
123 Grouse Family
    ruffed grouse
      (partridge)

124 Pheasant Family
  chicken
    eggs
  peafowl
  pheasant
  quail
125 Guinea Fowl Family
  guinea fowl
    eggs
126 Turkey Family
  turkey
    eggs
127 *Mammals*
128 Opossum Family
  opossum
129 Hare Family
  rabbit
130 Squirrel Family
  squirrel
131 Whale Family
  whale
132 Bear Family
  bear
133 Horse Family
  horse
134 Swine Family
  hog (pork)
    bacon
    ham
    lard
    pork gelatin
    sausage
    scrapple
135 Deer Family

  caribou
  deer (venison)
  elk
  moose
  reindeer
136 Pronghorn Family
  antelope
137 Bovine Family
  beef cattle
    beef
    beef by-products
      gelatin
      oleomargarine
      rennin (rennet)
      sausage casings
      suet
    milk products
      butter
      cheese
      ice cream
      lactose
      spray dried milk
      yogurt
    veal
  buffalo (bison)
  goat (kid)
    cheese
    ice cream
    milk
  sheep (domestic)
    lamb
    mutton
    Rocky Mountain sheep

Appendix B
Clinical Ecologists Practicing in a Controlled Environmental Hospital Setting

Physicians employing comprehensive environmental control, either in hospital units or in isolated rooms, include the following:

Argabrite, John W., M.D.
First National Bank Building
P.O. Box 258
Watertown, South Dakota 57201

Brooks, Clifton R., M.D., M.P.H
17400 W. Irvine Boulevard
Tustin, California 92680

Bullock, Thurman M., Jr., M.D.
722 N. Brown Street
Chadbourn, North Carolina 28431

Carroll, F. Murray, M.D.
722 N. Brown Street
Chadbourn, North Carolina 28431

Gerdes, Kendall A., M.D.
Presbyterian Hospital
1719 East 19th Avenue
Denver, Colorado 80218

Hosen, Harris, M.D.
2649 Proctor Street
Port Arthur, Texas 77640

Jackson, A. Verne, D.O.
1825 Maple Street
Forest Grove, Oregon 97116

Kroker, George F., M.D.
505 North Lake Shore Drive
Chicago, Illinois 60611

Marshall, Robert T., M.D.
505 North Lake Shore Drive
Chicago, Illinois 60611

Morgan, Joseph T., M.D.
Bay Clinic
1750 Thompson Road
Coos Bay, Oregon 97420

Peters, Dale W., M.D.
3201 East Second
Wichita, Kansas 67208

Randolph, Theron G., M.D.
505 North Lake Shore Drive
Chicago, Illinois 60611

Rea, William J., M.D.
8345 Walnut Hill Lane, Suite 240
Dallas, Texas 75231

Smiley, Ralph E., M.D.
8345 Walnut Hill Lane, Suite 240
Dallas, Texas 75231

Stroud, Robert M., M.D.
8345 Walnut Hill Lane, Suite 240
Dallas, Texas 75231

Appendix C
Sources of Further
Information

The following organizations can provide additional details concerning allergies and the field of clinical ecology:

Allergy Foundation of Lancaster County
Box 1424, Lancaster, Pennsylvania 17604
A nonprofit organization dedicated to furthering the understanding and treatment of allergic-type diseases. Publishes the works of Stephen D. Lockey, M.D. Write for information.

Human Ecology Action League (HEAL)
505 North Lake Shore Drive
Suite 6506
Chicago, Illinois 60611
A nationwide organization which fights for the rights and interests of patients and physicians in the field of environmental health. Publishes a newsletter. Write for information.

Human Ecology Research Foundation
505 North Lake Shore Drive
Suite 6506
Chicago, Illinois 60611
Supports research and publications in the field of clinical ecology. Source of reprints of the work of Dr. Theron G. Randolph, and of Dr. Randolph's bibliography. Publishes periodic bulletins as well as an annual report. Write for details.

Alan Mandell Center for Bio-Ecologic Diseases
3 Brush Street
Norwalk, Connecticut 06850

A nonprofit organization devoted to research, education, and treatment of ecologic disease. Has reprinted *Food Allergy* by Rinkel, Randolph, and Zeller, as well as papers by Dr. Marshall Mandell. Write for information.

Society for Clinical Ecolcgy
Del Stigler, M.D., Secretary
1750 Humboldt Street
Denver, Colorado 80218

A society of physicians, scientists, and other professionals dedicated to the investigation of chemical susceptibility and food allergy. Holds meetings, conducts basic and advanced seminars, and publishes archives. The Society can provide names of clinical ecologists in various parts of the United States and abroad.

Human Ecology Foundation (Toronto)
R.R. #1, Goodwood, Ontario
Canada LOC IAO

Suggested Reading

Carson, Rachel. *Silent Spring*. Boston: Houghton Mifflin, 1962. (A classic of the environmentalist movement)

Crook, William G. *Can Your Child Read? Is He Hyperactive?* Jackson, Tenn.: Pedicenter Press, 1975. (Readable guide for parents by a pediatrician/clinical ecologist)

———. *Tracking Down Hidden Food Allergies*. Jackson, Tenn.: Professional Books, 1978. (Elimination diets for diagnosis of food allergies)

Dickey, Lawrence, ed. *Clinical Ecology*. Springfield, Ill.: Charles C Thomas, 1970. (Medical textbook with eighty articles on the field by over forty experts)

Epstein, Samuel S. *The Politics of Cancer*. San Francisco: Sierra Books, 1979. (No mention of clinical ecology, but worth reading for data on spread and influence of chemical industry)

Forman, Robert. *How to Control Your Allergies*. New York: Larchmont Books, 1979. (Well-written introduction to the field in layman's terms)

Golos, Natalie; and Golbitz, Frances Golos, with Leighton, Frances Spatz. *Coping with Your Allergies*. New York: Simon and Schuster, 1979. (Comprehensive practical guide for the patient with food and chemical susceptibility)

Hunter, Beatrice Trum. *Consumer, Beware*. New York: Simon and Schuster, 1971. (A penetrating analysis of how our food supply has been adulterated and its nutrients lost)

———. *Mirage of Safety: Food Additives and Federal Policy*. New York: Charles Scribner's Sons, 1976.

Mackarness, Richard. *Eating Dangerously: The Hazards of Hidden Allergies*. New York and London: Harcourt Brace Jovanovich, 1976. (A British psychiatrist's popular account of the food allergy problem)

Mandell, Marshall, and Scanlon, Lynne Waller. *Dr. Mandell's 5-Day Allergy Relief System*. New York: Thomas Y. Crowell, 1979. (Self-help guide for environmental problems)

Moss, Ralph W. *The Cancer Syndrome*. New York: Grove Press, 1980. (Explains the difficulties often faced by medical innovators)

Randolph, Theron G. *Human Ecology and Susceptibility to the Chemical Environment*. Springfield, Ill.: Charles C Thomas, 1962 (sixth printing, 1978). (Comprehensive discussion of most aspects of the chemical-susceptibility problem)

Rapp, Doris J. *Allergies and the Hyperactive Child*. New York: Sovereign, 1979. (Pertinence of clinical ecology to children by a prominent Buffalo, New York, pediatrician)

Rinkel, H. J.; Randolph, T. G.; and Zeller, M. *Food Allergy*. Norwalk, Conn.: New England Foundation of Allergic and Environmental Diseases (reprinted 1951). (Classic textbook on the subject)

Notes

INTRODUCTION: Dr. Randolph's Alternative

. 1. Theron G. Randolph, M.D., *Testimony in the Matter of a Definition and Standard of Identity for Bread and Related Products*, Washington, D.C., Docket No. FDC–31 (B), Before the Administrator, Federal Security Agency, August 3, 1949, pp. 14593–14628.

2. United States Department of Commerce, Bureau of the Census. "Current Industrial Reports: Pharmaceutical Preparations, Except Biologicals." Washington, D.C., 1977, p. 3.

3. For another such case see: Doris J. Rapp, M.D., "Double-blind Confirmation and Treatment of Milk Sensitivity," *Med. J. Aust.*, 1978, 1:571–572.

CHAPTER 1: Hidden Addictions

1. Edward M. Brecher and the Editors of Consumer Reports, *Licit and Illicit Drugs* (Boston: Little, Brown and Company, 1972), p. 205. Excellent discussion of caffeine as an abused drug.

2. Nils Bejerot, *Addiction and Society* (Springfield, Ill.: Charles C Thomas, 1970), p. 23.

3. Theron G. Randolph, "Biographical Sketch of Herbert J. Rinkel, M.D., Emphasizing His Medical Contributions," in *Allergy: Including IgE in Diagnosis and Treatment*, ed. Fordyce Johnson, M.D. (Chicago: Year Book Medical Publishers, 1979).

4. This is a fictitious name. All of the cases discussed in this book are those of real people whom I have treated, and whose stories are recorded in my medical records. The medical facts are true, but the names and sometimes other circumstantial details have been changed to protect these patients' anonymity.

5. Brecher et al., *op. cit.*

6. Marshall Mandell, M.D., and Lynn Waller Scanlon, *Dr. Mandell's 5-Day Allergy Relief System* (New York: Thomas Y. Crowell, 1979).

7. Arthur F. Coca, M.D., *Familial Nonreaginic Food Allergy* (Springfield, Ill.: Charles C Thomas, 1945).

CHAPTER 2: The Ups and Downs of Addicted Life

1. Paul H. Wender, M.D., *Minimal Brain Dysfunction in Children* (New York: Wiley-Interscience, 1971).

2. Theron G. Randolph, M.D., "Adaptation to Specific Environmental Exposures Enhanced by Individual Susceptibility," in *Clinical Ecology*, Lawrence D. Dickey, M.D., ed. (Springfield, Ill.: Charles C Thomas, 1976), p. 46.

3. Theron G. Randolph, M.D., "Specific Adaptation," *Ann. Allergy*, 40:333–345, May 1978.

4. E. F. Adolph, "General and Specific Characteristics of Physiological Adaptation," *Am. J. Physiol.*, 184:18, 1956.

5. Hans Selye, M.D., "The General Adaptation Syndrome and the Diseases of Adaptation," *J. Allergy*, 17:231–247, 289–323, 358–398, 1946.

6. Hans Selye, M.D., *Stress* (Montreal: Acta, 1950).

7. D. B. Dill, E. F. Adolph, and C. G. Wilber, *Handbook of Physiology, Adaptation to the Environment* (Washington, D.C.: American Physiological Society, 1964).

8. Iris R. Bell, Ph.D., M.D., "A Kinin Model of Mediation for Food and Chemical Sensitivities; Biobehavioral Implications," *Ann. Allergy*, 35:206–215, 1975.

9. Theron G. Randolph, M.D., "The Alternation of the Symptoms of Allergy and Those of Alcoholism and Certain Mental Disturbances," *J. Lab. & Clin. Med.*, 40:932, 1952.

10. George H. Savage, M.D., *Insanity and Allied Neuroses* (Philadelphia: Henry C. Lea's & Company, 1884).

11. C. Orian Truss, M.D., "Tissue Injury Induced by Candida Albicans; Mental and Neurological Manifestations," *Orthomolecular Psychiatry*, 7:17–37, 1978.

CHAPTER 3: The Problem of Chemical Susceptibility

1. Theron G. Randolph, M.D., *Human Ecology and Susceptibility to the Chemical Environment* (Springfield, Ill.: Charles C Thomas, 1962).

2. Sameul S. Epstein, *The Politics of Cancer* (San Francisco: Sierra Club Books, 1978), p. 34.

CHAPTER 4: The Chemicals in Our Food

1. Epstein, *op. cit.*

2. Philip M. Boffey, "Death of a Dye," *New York Times Magazine*, February 29, 1976.

3. Stephen D. Lockey, M.D., "Sensitivity to F.D. & C. Dyes in Drugs, Foods and Beverages," in *Clinical Ecology*, ed. Lawrence D. Dickey, M.D. (Springfield, Ill.: Charles C Thomas, 1976), pp. 334–342.

4. T. G. Randolph, M.D., and J. P. Rollins, M.D., "Allergic Reactions from Ingestion or Intravenous Injection of Cane Sugar (Sucrose)," *J. Lab. & Clin. Med.*, 36:242–248, Aug., 1950.

5. Epstein, *op. cit.*

6. James Ridgeway, *The Politics of Ecology* (New York: E. P. Dutton & Co., Inc., 1970), p. 35.

7. S. H. Watson and C. S. Kibler, "Drinking Water as a Cause of Asthma," *J. Allergy*, 5:197, 1934.

CHAPTER 5: The Dangers of Drugs, Cosmetics, and Perfumes

1. United States Department of Commerce, *op. cit.*

2. Stephen D. Lockey, M.D., "Reactions to Hidden Drugs," in *Clinical Ecology*, ed. Lawrence D. Dickey, M.D. (Springfield, Ill.: Charles C Thomas, 1976), pp. 343–347.

3. Stephen D. Lockey, M.D., "Sensitivity to F.D. & C. Dyes in Drugs, Foods and Beverages," in Dickey, *op. cit.*, p. 335.

4. Jerome Glaser, M.D., *Allergy in Childhood* (Springfield, Ill.: Charles C Thomas, 1956).

CHAPTER 6: Indoor Air Pollution

1. Guy O. Pfeiffer, M.D., and Casimir M. Nikel, F.A.C.H.A., eds., *The Household Environment and Chronic Illness—Guidelines for Constructing and Maintaining a Less Polluted Residence* (Springfield, Ill.: Charles C Thomas, 1980). This book contains detailed information on many aspects of the indoor air pollution problem.

2. See Mandell and Scanlon, *op. cit.*, pp. 203–210, for a good popular discussion of this problem.

3. Natalie Golos and Frances Golos Golbitz with Frances Spatz Leighton, *Coping with Your Allergies* (New York: Simon and Schuster, 1979), contains a wealth of practical information on where and how to find alternative materials.

4. Alsoph H. Corwin, Ph.D., "Ozone," in Lawrence D. Dickey, M.D., *op. cit.*, pp. 285–291.

5. *The Washington Post*, March 25, 1980.

6. Copies of this report, *Air Pollution in Schools and Its Effect on Our Children*, are available from the Human Ecology Research Foundation, 505 North Lakeshore Drive, Chicago, Illinois 60611. Prices on request.

7. *Ibid.* Contains a discussion of this problem and refers to the work of Dr. Angus L. MacLean of the Johns Hopkins University, which was published in the *Transactions of the American Academy of Ophthalmology and Otolaryngology*, 1967.

8. *Ibid.* A personal communication to Mrs. Blume.

9. Claudia S. Miller, "Mass Psychogenic Illness or Chemically-Induced Hypersusceptibility?" Prepared for the symposium "The Diagnosis and Amelioration of Mass Psychogenic Illness" and sponsored by the U.S. Department of Health, Education, and Welfare, National Institute for Occupational Safety and Health, Chicago, Illinois, May 30–June 1, 1979.

CHAPTER 7: Outdoor Air Pollution

1. Golos et al., *op. cit.*, pp. 261–271, contains practical information for the susceptible traveler.

2. *New York Times*, May 27, 1979.

CHAPTER 8: Levels of Reaction in Environmental Disease

1. Theron G. Randolph, M.D., C. Richard Ahroon, M.D., Harry G. Clark, M.D., George S. Frauenberger, M.D., J. Interlandi, M.D., Donald S. Mitchell, M.D., Ralph C. Roberts, M.D., Robert P. Watterson, M.D., and Hugo Zotter, M.D., "Specific Adaptive Illness," 112th Annual Meeting of the American Psychiatric Association, Chicago, Illinois, May 1956, and the 105th Annual Meeting of the American Medical Association, Chicago, Illinois, June 1956.

CHAPTER 9: Hyperactivity (Plus-two Reaction)

1. Doris J. Rapp, M.D., "Does Diet Affect Hyperactivity?" *Journal of Learning Disabilities*, Volume 11, Number 6, June/July 1978, provides an excellent overview of this problem.

2. Theron G. Randolph, M.D., "Allergy as a Causative Factor in Fatigue, Irritability and Behavior Problems in Children," *J. Pediat.*, 1947, 31:560–572.

3. Benjamin Feingold, *Why Your Child is Hyperactive* (New York: Random House, 1974). See Mandell and Scanlon, *op. cit.*, pp. 138–141, for a critique of Feingold's theories from the point of view of clinical ecology.

4. *Business Week*, December 17, 1979.

5. *Ibid.*

CHAPTER 10: Alcoholism (Plus-two Reaction)

1. Theron G. Randolph, M.D., "The Mechanism of Chronic Alcoholism," *J. Lab. & Clin. Med.*, 36:978, December, 1950 (abstract).

2. Theron G. Randolph, M.D., "Descriptive Features of Food Addiction; Addictive Eating and Drinking," *Quart. J. Studies Alcohol*, 17:195–224, 1956.

3. Richard Mackarness, "The Allergic Factor in Alcoholism," *International Journal of Social Psychiatry*, Autumn, 1972, page 194.

4. Marshall Mandell, M.D., and Lynne Waller Scanlon, *op. cit.*, pp. 114–132.

5. Theron G. Randolph, M.D., "The Role of Specific Alcoholic Beverages," in Dickey, ed., *op. cit.*, pp. 321–333.

CHAPTER 12: Headache (Minus-two Reaction)

1. Francis Hare, M.D., *The Food Factor in Disease*, vols. I and II (London: Longmans, 1905).

2. Albert H. Rowe, M.D., "Food Allergy, a Common Cause of Abdominal Symptoms and Headache," Food Facts 3:7, 1927.

3. Warren T. Vaughan, M.D., "Allergic Migraine," *J. Amer. Med. Assn.*, 88:1383, 1927.

4. J. M. Sheldon, M.D., and T. G. Randolph, M.D., "Allergy in Migraine-like Headaches," *Am. J. Med. Sc.*, 190:232–237, Aug., 1935.

CHAPTER 13: Arthritis and Related Muscle and Joint Pains

1. Michael Zeller, M.D., "Rheumatoid Arthritis—Food Allergy as a Factor," *Ann. Allergy*, 7:200–205, 1949.
2. Herbert J. Rinkel, M.D., Theron G. Randolph, M.D., and Michael Zeller, M.D., *Food Allergy* (Springfield, Ill.: Charles C Thomas, 1951).
3. Theron G. Randolph, M.D. "Ecologically Oriented Rheumatoid Arthritis," in Dickey, ed., *op. cit.*, pp. 201–212.
4. Theron G. Randolph, M.D., "Allergic Myalgia," *J. Mich. Med. Soc.*, 50:487–494, May, 1951.

CHAPTER 14: Fatigue (Minus-two Reaction) and Brain-fag (Minus-three Reaction)

1. A. H. Rowe, M.D., "Allergic Toxemia and Migraine Due to Food Allergy," *Calif. West. Med.*, 33:785, 1930.
2. Theron G. Randolph, M.D., "Fatigue and Weakness of Allergic Origin (Allergic Toxemia) To Be Differentiated from 'Nervous Fatigue' or Neurasthenia," *Ann. Allergy*, 3:418–430, November–December, 1945.
3. Arthur F. Coca, M.D., *op. cit.*
4. Theron G. Randolph, M.D., "Allergic Ills Limiting Student Performance," Procedures of 29th Annual Meeting, American College Health Association, 31:46–48, 1951.

CHAPTER 15: Depression (Minus-three and Minus-four Reactions)

1. Theron G. Randolph, M.D., "An Experimentally Induced Acute Psychotic Episode Following the Intubation of an Allergenic Food," 7th Annual Congress, American College of Allergists, Chicago, Illinois, February, 1951.
2. Theron G. Randolph, M.D., "Allergic Factors in the Etiology of Certain Mental Symptoms," *J. Lab. and Clin. Med.*, 36:977, 1950.
3. Theron G. Randolph, M.D., "Depressions Caused by Home Exposures to Gas and Combustion Products of Gas, Oil and Coal," *J. Lab. and Clin. Med.*, 46:942, 1955.
4. Theron G. Randolph, M.D., "Ecologic Mental Illness—Psychiatry Exteriorized," *J. Lab. and Clin. Med.*, 54:936, 1959.
5. F. C. Donan, "Cereals and Schizophrenia," *Acta Psychiatrica Scandinavica*, 42:125–152, 1966.
6. F. C. Donan, M.D., J. C. Grasberger, M.D., F. M. Lowell, M.D., et al., "Relapsed Schizophrenics: More Rapid Improvements on a Milk and Cereal-Free Diet," *British J. Psychiatry*, 115:585–596, 1969.
7. Frederic Speer, M.D., ed., *Allergy of the Nervous System* (Springfield, Ill.: Charles C Thomas, 1970).
8. Richard Mackarness, M.D., *Eating Dangerously* (New York and London: Harcourt Brace Jovanovich, 1976). Published in England under the title of *Not All in the Mind* (London: Pan Ltd., 1976).
9. Marshall Mandell, M.D., and Lynne W. Scanlon, *Dr. Mandell's 5-Day Allergy Relief System* (New York: Thomas Y. Crowell, 1979).
10. Richard Mackarness, M.D., *Chemical Victims* (London: Pan Ltd., 1980).
11. William H. Philpott, M.D., and Dwight K. Kalida, *Brain Allergy—The Psychonutrient Connection* (New Haven: Keats, 1980).

CHAPTER 16: Interviews and In-Office Procedures

1. C. H. Lee, M.D., and H. J. Rinkel, M.D., "A New Test for the Detection of Food Allergies and Pollen and Mold Incompatibility," *Trans. Soc. Ophthalmol. Otolaryngol. Allergy*, 3:1, 1962.
2. A. H. Rowe, M.D., *Clinical Allergy* (Philadelphia: Lea and Febiger, 1937).

3. Herbert J. Rinkel, M.D., cited in Rinkel, Randolph, and Zeller, *op. cit.*, pp. 144–147.

4. Theron G. Randolph, M.D., "The Provocative Hydrocarbon Test," *J. Lab. and Clin. Med.*, 64:995, 1964.

5. Harris Hosen, M.D., "Hydrocarbons and Other Gases, As Related to the Field of Allergy," in Dickey, ed., *op. cit.*, pp. 262–268.

CHAPTER 17: The Ecology Unit

1. Theron G. Randolph, M.D., "Ecologic Orientation in Medicine; Comprehensive Environmental Control in Diagnosis and Therapy," *Ann. Allergy*, 23:7–22, 1965.

2. Dickey, ed., *op. cit.*, p. 69.

3. A compatible water may not be found: We test routinely and blindly with seven different waters; there are about a dozen others that we have available and use if we cannot find a compatible source. See also Theron G. Randolph, M.D., *Human Ecology and Susceptibility to the Chemical Environment*.

4. Dickey, ed., *op. cit.*, pp. 577–597.

CHAPTER 18: Coping with Food Allergies: The Rotary Diversified Diet

1. Herbert J. Rinkel, M.D., "Food Allergy, IV: The Function and Clinical Application of the Rotary Diversified Diet," *J. Pediat.*, 32:266, 1948.

2. Rinkel, Randolph, and Zeller, *op. cit.*, p. 238.

3. Theron G. Randolph, M.D., "The Role of Specific Sugars," in Dickey, ed., *op. cit.*, pp. 310–320.

4. Theron G. Randolph, M.D., "Biologic Dietetics," in Dickey, ed., *op. cit.*, pp. 107–122.

CHAPTER 19: The Chemical Questionnaire

1. Cited in Golos et al., *op. cit.*, p. 53.

2. Joseph F. Fraumeni, Jr., ed. *Persons at High Risk of Cancer* (New York: Academic Press, 1975).

3. Guy O. Pfeiffer, M.D., "Environmental Hazards in the Office," in Dickey, ed., *op. cit.*, pp. 367–368.

CHAPTER 20: Coping with Chemical Exposure

1. George E. Delury, ed., *The World Almanac and Book of Facts, 1980* (New York: Newspaper Enterprise Association, 1979), p. 954.

2. Mandell and Scanlon, *op. cit.*, p. 188.

3. *Ibid.*, p. 189.

4. *Ibid.*, p. 87n.

CHAPTER 21: Clinical Ecology Versus Conventional Medicine

1. Delury, ed., *op. cit.*, p. 957.

2. *Ibid.*, pp. 957–958.

3. Paul H. Wender, *Minimal Brain Dysfunction in Children* (New York: Wiley-Interscience, 1971).

4. Harry Milt, *Serious Mental Illness in Children* (New York: Public Affairs Pamphlet #352, November, 1974).

5. Theodore Irwin, *Depression: Causes and Treatment* (New York: Public Affairs Pamphlet #488, January, 1973).

6. Ronald R. Fieve, *Moodswing: The Third Revolution in Psychiatry* (New York: Bantam Books, 1976).

7. Milt, *op. cit.*

8. *The Problem of Mental Retardation*, DHEW Pub. No. (OHI) 75–22003 (Washington, D.C.: Department of Health, Education and Welfare, 1975).

9. Heywood Gould, *Headaches and Health* (New York: St. Martin's Press, 1972), pp. 2–3.

11. Dr. John E. Bulette, psychiatrist at the Medical College of Pennsylvania, quoted in *U.S. News and World Report*, May 14, 1979, p. 27.

12. Brecher et al., *op. cit.*

13. Howard G. Rapaport and Shirley Motter Linde, *The Complete Allergy Guide* (New York: Simon and Schuster, 1970).

14. Delury, *op. cit.*, p. 953.

15. *Ibid.*, p. 959.

16. U.S. Department of Commerce, *op. cit.*

17. *Ibid.*

18. Joseph Kett, *The Formation of the American Medical Profession: The Role of Institutions, 1780–1860* (New Haven: Yale University Press, 1968).

19. But see Harvey W. Wiley, M.D., *The History of a Crime Against the Food Law* (Milwaukee: Lee Foundation for Nutritional Research, 1955 [1929]), by the first commissioner of the Food and Drug Administration, who claimed that the laws were "perverted to protect adulteration of foods and drugs."

Index